Contents

· Contributors ·

Jack B. Anon, M.D., F.A.C.S., F.A.A.O.A.
Clinical Assistant Professor
Department of Otolaryngology
University of Pittsburgh Medical Center
Pittsburgh, Pennsylvania

Private Practice
Erie, Pennsylvania

B. Jane Dixon, B.S., F.A.A.O.A.
Head, Allergy Department
Dixon Medical Center
Rome, Georgia

Hamilton S. Dixon, M.D., F.A.A.O.A.
Assistant Clinical Professor
Department of Otolaryngology
Vanderbilt University
Nashville, Tennessee

Private Practice
Rome, Georgia

Joseph P. Keenan, M.D., F.A.C.S., F.A.A.O.A.
Assistant Clinical Professor
Department of Surgery
University of Connecticut Medical School
Farmington, Connecticut

Active Staff
Noble Hospital
Westfield, Massachussetts

Hueston C. King, M.D., F.A.C.S., F.A.A.O.A.
Clinical Associate Professor
Department of Otolaryngology
University of Texas Southwestern Medical Center
Dallas, Texas

Private Practice
Venice, Florida

William P. King, M.D., F.A.C.S., F.A.A.O.A.
Clinical Assistant Professor
Department of Otorhinolaryngology
Baylor College of Medicine
Houston, Texas

Private Practice
Corpus Christi, Texas

Helen F. Krause, M.D., F.A.C.S., F.A.A.O.A.
Associate Clinical Professor
Department of Otolaryngology
University of Pittsburgh Medical Center

Private Practice
Pittsburgh, Pennsylvania

Richard L. Mabry, M.D., F.A.C.S., F.A.A.O.A.
Professor
Department of Otorhinolaryngology
University of Texas Southwestern Medical Center
Dallas, Texas

Walter A. Ward, M.D., P.A., F.A.A.O.A.
Private Practice
Winston-Salem, North Carolina

· *Preface to the Second Edition* ·

I am pleased to be the series editor for the American Academy of Otolaryngic Allergy monographs. The second edition of *Skin Endpoint Titration* has been reviewed by the AAOA Medical Education Committee and updated with an eye to the new regulations from OSHA and CLIA. While these are always changing, updating texts to include these important safeguards for our patients and ourselves will improve our medical care. The text remains a classic reference for continuing education in otolaryngic allergy.

Jacquelynne P. Corey, M.D., F.A.C.S., F.A.A.O.A.

· *Preface to the First Edition* ·

Despite continuing advances in the diagnosis of immunoglobulin E (IgE)-mediated inhalant allergy utilizing *in vitro* technology, the otolaryngic allergist should be familiar with the principles and practice of skin endpoint titration (SET). Even if SET is not the practitioner's primary testing modality, familiarity with skin testing techniques and responses will allow proper interpretation of *in vitro*-based antigen vial tests, will permit the blending of *in vitro* and *in vivo* test methods within an allergy practice, and will often "bail out" the practitioner caught in a confusing situation.

This monograph is provided as a convenient introduction and reference source. It should also be useful in preparing for the Fellowship examination of the American Academy of Otolaryngic Allergy (AAOA). However, simply studying this material will not prepare an individual to practice SET. The person undertaking the practice of otolaryngic allergy is advised to attend an AAOA-sponsored basic course in otolaryngic allergy and to upgrade their proficiency further by taking advantage of AAOA-sponsored advanced courses as well as AAOA meeting presentations and instruction courses, and other opportunities for further education in this ever-expanding and complex field.

I would like to express my appreciation to each author for his or her contribution, not only as tangibly manifested by the chapters they have prepared, but in their involvement in the teaching efforts of the AAOA. The publication of this monograph by Thieme Medical Publishers marks a milestone in the continuing educational activities of the AAOA. Other volumes will follow, and we hope you will find each of them useful in your practice of otolaryngic allergy.

Richard L. Mabry, M.D., F.A.C.S., F.A.A.O.A.

· 1 ·

Preparing to Do Skin Endpoint Titration in an Office Setting

HELEN F. KRAUSE, M.D., F.A.C.S., F.A.A.O.A.

The basic requirements necessary to add allergy to an otolaryngology practice are training, personnel, and the actual office set-up including space, equipment, and supplies. Some time will have to be allotted to activate this portion of your practice and to control it.

Training

Just as in learning to do a new surgical procedure, proper training is essential. For otolaryngic allergy this may include:

1. AAOA basic courses—one or more.
2. AAOA advanced courses—one or more.
3. AAOA scientific programs—at annual and interim meetings.
4. Instruction courses—at the annual meeting.
5. Fellowships and preceptorships—varying programs are available.
6. Continuing review of allergy literature.
7. Review of videotapes on skin endpoint titration (SET) and radioallergosorbent test (RAST) (available for purchase from the AAOA).
8. Further professional advancement through achieving Fellowship status.

Personnel

The personnel you hire to work with allergy patients must be well trained. You will need at least one assistant. As the practice develops, more may be needed. Some physicians use in-office personnel; others may hire and train new assistants. The allergy assistant may be a registered nurse (RN), a licensed practical nurse (LPN), a medical assistant, a physician's assistant, a medical technician, or a technologist.

The allergy assistant must be interested and enthusiastic. The physician, however, must take the ultimate responsibility for the allergy practice. Employees cannot be sent to courses alone and be expected to return to be the office allergist. If an employee leaves abruptly it will be up to the physician to provide on-the-job training until the replacement can be formally trained at a course. This is only possible if the physician is familiar with day-to-day operation of the allergy practice.

Secretarial assistance is necessary, although initially you may need only a part-time secretary or use your general office secretary. Eventually, however, you will need full-time help in this portion of your practice. A secretary to do the special bookkeeping necessary for an allergy practice may require separate space and possibly a special allergy patient filing system. The practice of allergy involves many small charges and considerable specialized insurance processing. If your office is computerized, a special program may be required that differs from your routine otolaryngology procedures.

As your allergy practice grows, you may elect to hire personnel whose primary function will be separate from the clinical otolaryngology practice.

Customizing an Otolaryngic Allergy Office

An allergy section can be incorporated into an established otolaryngology practice (Fig. 1-1). It is important to allot a separate space initially, even if only a small one is available. An average examining room is usually sufficient. As you expand your practice you may need to contemplate acquiring additional room. Storage space is a must. Supplies such as syringes and bottles will be most economically purchased in bulk and they will have to be stored as the practice grows.

The allergy patient will be initially evaluated in most offices as a general otolaryngology patient. If the appointment secretary can be trained to recognize patients with possible allergic problems, a special allergy questionnaire can be sent to be completed and returned to the office or brought in for the first appointment. This can save a considerable amount of time in history taking. A questionnaire supplemented by an individual history should always be completed before allergy testing, to aid in selection of the proper antigens for testing.

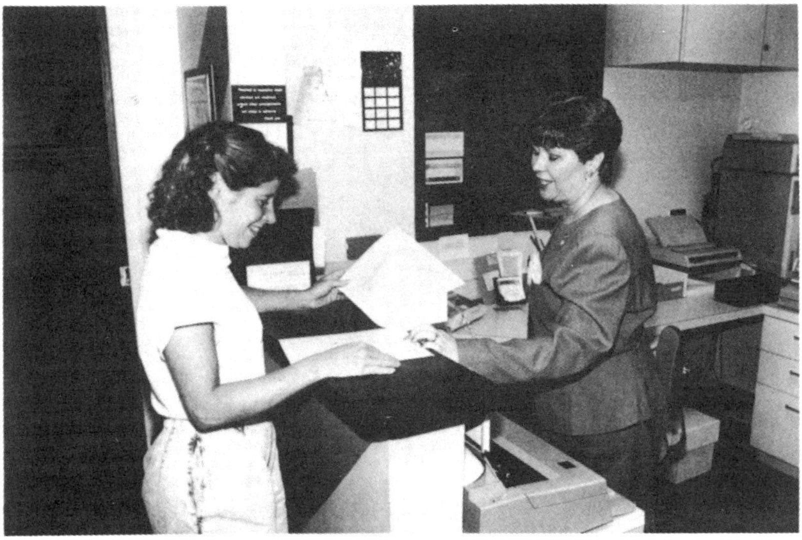

Figure 1-1. The receptionist registers the patient and explains the allergy questionnaire before the patient is seen by the doctor.

Testing and Treatment Area

Some physicians prefer individual rooms to test patients, providing privacy for the patient and preventing confusion. Many doctors do not find these a necessity, and are comfortable with an open area, allowing one nurse to observe several patients. Space should also be available for a patient to lie down in case of vasovagal or true anaphylactic reactions. For this, some allergists use a folding cot, others a couch or a reclining chair.

Although patients should be instructed to wear short-sleeved shirts for testing, it is well to have jackets or gowns available.

The treatment area should be able to accommodate several patients. The testing area may be used to give treatment injections during scheduled "shot hours" (Fig. 1-2). It is valuable, if the office arrangement permits, to have a separate waiting area for a few allergy patients apart from the general otolaryngology area for better control of patient flow and observation for reactions (Fig. 1-3).

Ideally, the allergy assistant should have a private area to present pretest information and forms, hold conferences when necessary, answer phone questions, and do chart work.

For the space allotted for allergy you will need to select furniture, including some special allergy equipment. First, a chair to test the patient: an examining chair is acceptable but it is easier to use a higher and smaller chair. A

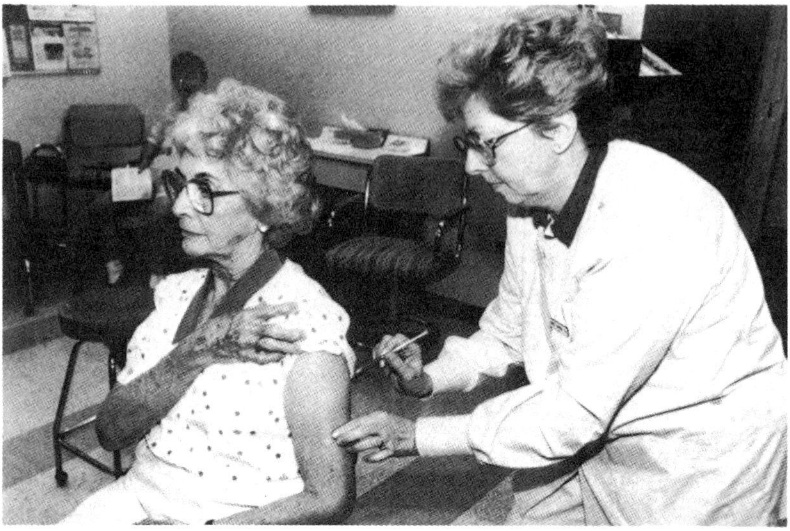

Figure 1-2. A combined testing and treatment room is adequate. Proper technique must be maintained in giving allergy injections using the posterolateral aspect of the arm, carefully aspirating before injection.

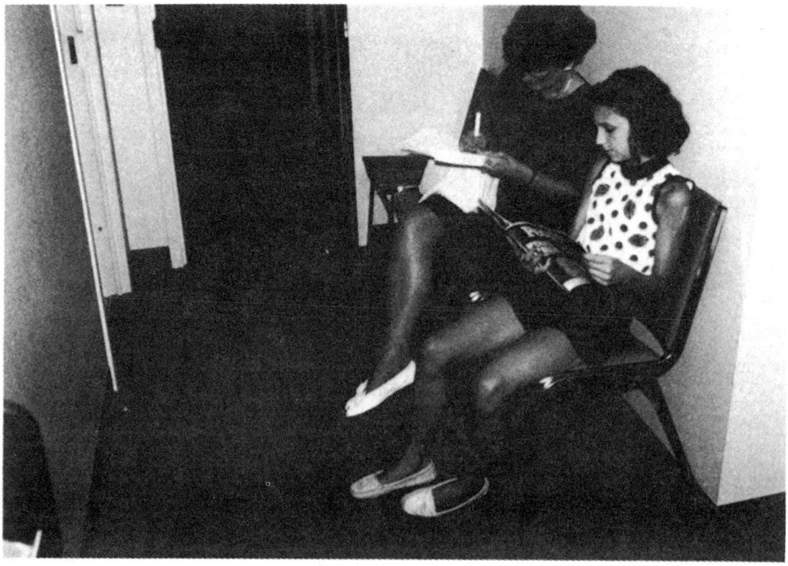

Figure 1-3. A separate entrance and waiting area for allergy patients improves traffic flow and patient management.

comfortable bar stool with arms works well. The tester should have a chair or stool on wheels positioned to place him or her slightly lower than the patient's chair. Some assistants like a back support, others do not. A cart, cabinet, or counter of proper height is necessary to hold testing materials, with shelves or drawers for storage of emergency supplies. Be sure everyone knows where the emergency supplies are and keep them up to date with fresh batteries, and so forth (Fig. 1-4). In addition, be sure all personnel are familiar with emergency protocol, including cardiopulmonary resuscitation (CPR). Although systemic reactions are rarely encountered with skin endpoint titration or immunotherapy they present a potential hazard. Also plan to provide reading materials, including educational materials about allergy. Toys or games to occupy the children and small gifts for the children are also desirable.

A laboratory is valuable but not essential. Tests performed may range from hemograms, monospot tests, and nasal cytology to *in vitro* immunoglobulin E (IgE) testing (Fig. 1-5). With newer technology, especially the enzyme and monoclonal antibody procedures, the equipment is small and the space and supplies required are minimal. You will need both counter and storage space. A reclining chair is excellent for venipunctures and for nervous patients.

There should be quiet space and time for mixing the testing and treatment boards and patient vials (Fig. 1-6). If these are not done accurately and on time a disaster could result. A good refrigerator is essential—the largest size your space will accommodate. If you plan to do *in vitro* testing, do not get a frost-free model (so frozen serum will not defrost) (Fig. 1-7).

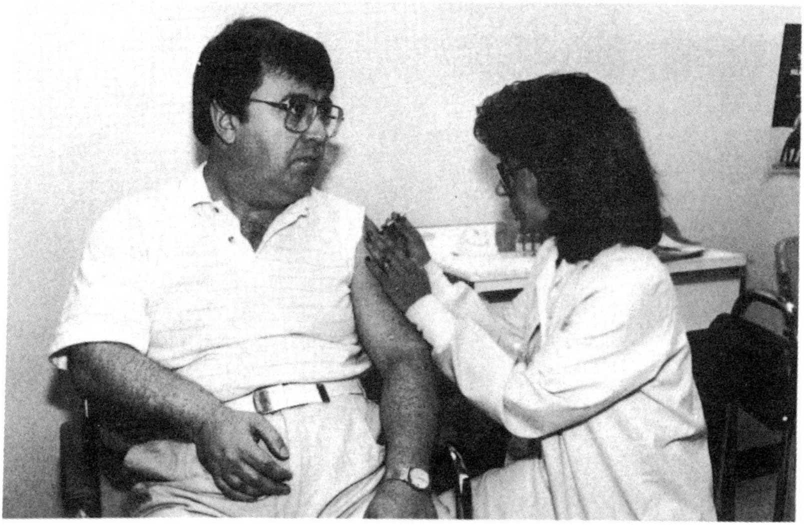

Figure 1-4. Proper technique for applying intradermal tests must be maintained with equipment and furniture in comfortable positions.

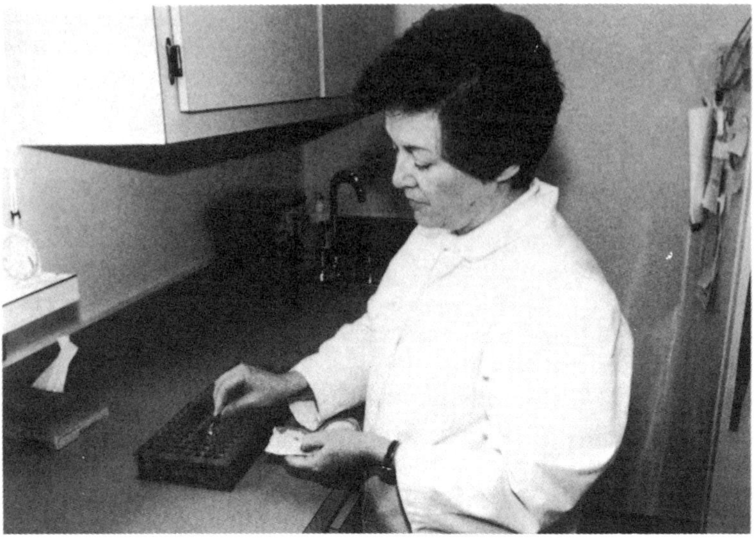

Figure 1-5. Various *in vitro* tests may be selected. Illustrated is disc loading into vials for a RAST process by the medical technologist. The sink used to prepare nasal cytology slides is to the right.

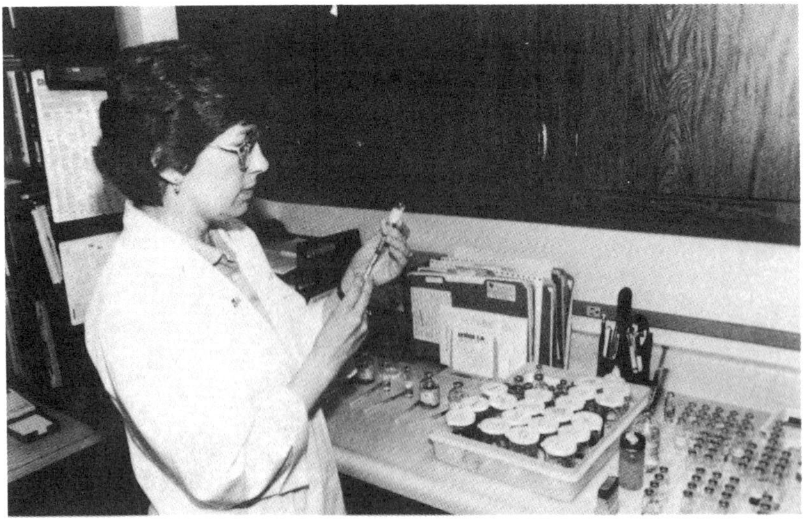

Figure 1-6. The allergy nurse prepares testing and treatment sets and patient vials, carefully controlling all steps.

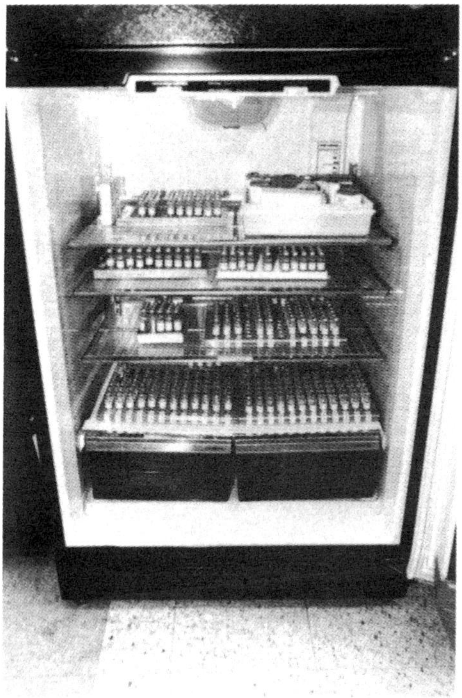

Figure 1-7. A large refrigerator is an important addition to an allergy practice.

Supplies

Specialized supplies will be needed for an allergy practice (Fig. 1-8). These include:

- sterilized bottles/vials.
- syringes and needles.
- vial racks.
- trays.
- cotton.
- rulers (metric).
- diluents.
- antigens.
- timers.
- alcohol containers.
- labels.
- forms.

Don't buy everything in sight. Start slowly and conservatively. Presterilized glass bottles or vials are available with fixed aluminum caps, empty or

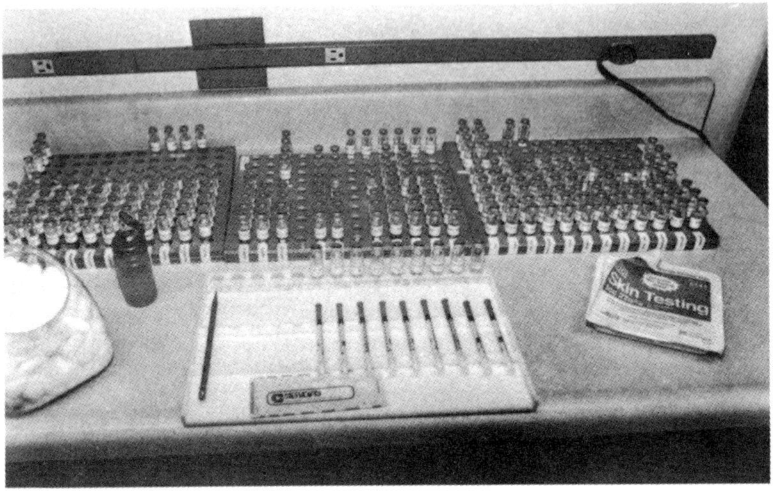

Figure 1-8. The equipment and materials must be prepared carefully before intradermal testing is begun: vials of diluted antigens in racks, proper testing syringes, cotton balls, alcohol, a measuring device, and a timer are necessary.

with premeasured volume of diluent in 5-cc or 10-cc sizes for testing and treatment sets and 1-cc, 5-cc, and 10-cc sizes for patient treatment vials. The size selected depends on the number of antigens being used and the number of injections per vial. Some doctors prefer 1-cc single-dose treatment bottles. All testing, stock treatment, and patient treatment vials must be properly labeled and dated.

Disposable syringes for allergy use are available from several companies. These are hubless, either 0.5 or 1.0 cc in size, with the needles attached to eliminate dead space and make dosage more accurate. Either the 0.5-cc or 1.0-cc size may be used for testing. The 1.0-cc size is most practical for treatment. There are also a variety of needle sizes (25–27 gauge) available for mixing, testing, and treatment. The most commonly used needles are 26- and 27-gauge ⅜″ with intradermal bevels for mixing and testing, and 27-gauge ⅜″ or ½″ with regular bevel for immunotherapy. Special packages are available for patient purchase with 10 1-cc syringes with 27-gauge ½″ needles. Proper containers to dispose of syringes and needles are essential in an office.

Racks are used to hold testing and treatment set bottles. Plastic racks are moisture-resistant and easier to clean than wood. They are available in a number of sizes to hold various sizes and number of vials. Be sure the racks you select will fit into your refrigerator. The rows should have six to eight holes to accommodate the 1:5 dilution bottles. It is convenient to have trays to hold filled testing syringes. Any type of convenient timer is acceptable. You will need containers for cotton and alcohol, and proper wheal-measuring rulers. You may want to use a skin marker initially if you are more comfortable identifying each test as it is applied.

Diluent may be purchased in bulk or in premeasured vials containing 4 cc or 8 cc. Diluents available are buffered phenolated saline, human serum albumin, or glycerinated saline. (For details, see Chapter 6 on vial preparation.)

Antigens are sold as concentrates, in 50% glycerine solution. Some are now standardized by allergy units; others are still sold as w/v in 1:10, 1:20, 1:33⅓, or 1:100 concentrations. Be aware of the concentration of each antigen in preparing your testing treatment boards. Order enough of the basic antigens you plan to use to last a year. Start with the inhalants and epidermals. As more standardized extracts become available, they will replace current products and will have to be worked into the practice with safety precautions.

Buy antigens most common in your area. As you identify more allergens that you might need, buy a small amount. If you use up each completely before it expires, you may want to add it to your permanent board and buy a larger bottle next time.

Initially, most otolaryngologists use dietary management for food allergy, so don't buy food antigens at first. Become comfortable with skin endpoint titration, then add food testing.

Forms

Allergy requires a considerable amount of paperwork. You should have a prepared statement of allergy concepts and your approach to testing and treatment for the patient. This may be given to the patient with the allergy questionnaire, which was mentioned earlier. Explain in writing your fee schedule and insurance policies. Patients should sign authorization forms for testing and treatment. Appointment cards with instructions on clothing to wear for testing and medication avoidance also should be given to the patient. The schedule for "shot hours" should be outlined and posted. Each patient should be told what is in each vial and the vial's cost (Fig. 1-9).

If the injections are to be given other than in your office (at another physician's office, a school, a work health facility, or by a nurse or other trained individual), very detailed instructions must be provided (Fig. 1-10). Reports of the results of the injections and of local or systemic reactions must be returned before new vials are made. Instruction material for the patient about environmental control is needed. The more that is given in writing to the patient, the more the patient will remember and the better compliance with treatment will be.

You must become familiar with current procedural terminology (CPT) codes (see Table 1-1), tables, and the policies of local insurance companies to be reimbursed properly. For example, in some states insurors will pay far less

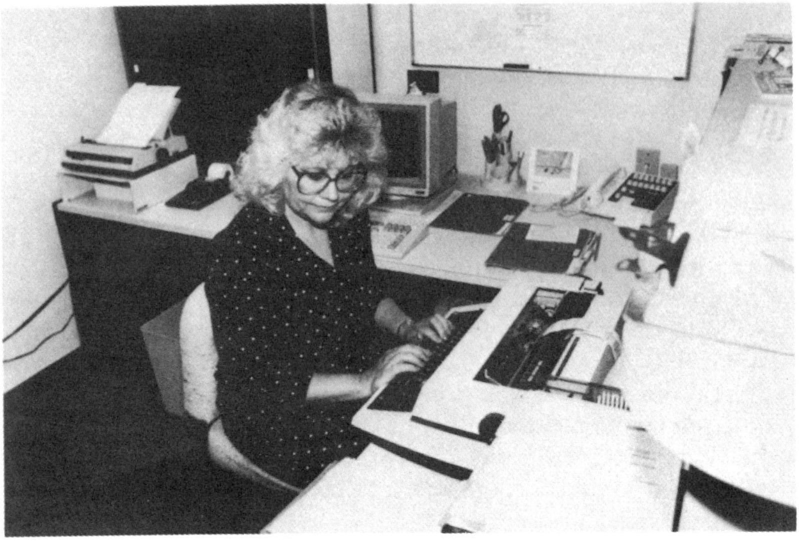

Figure 1-9. Secretary prepares vial labels and information for the patient about allergy testing, treatment, and cost. Special forms are prepared if the patient is to receive the injections outside the allergy office.

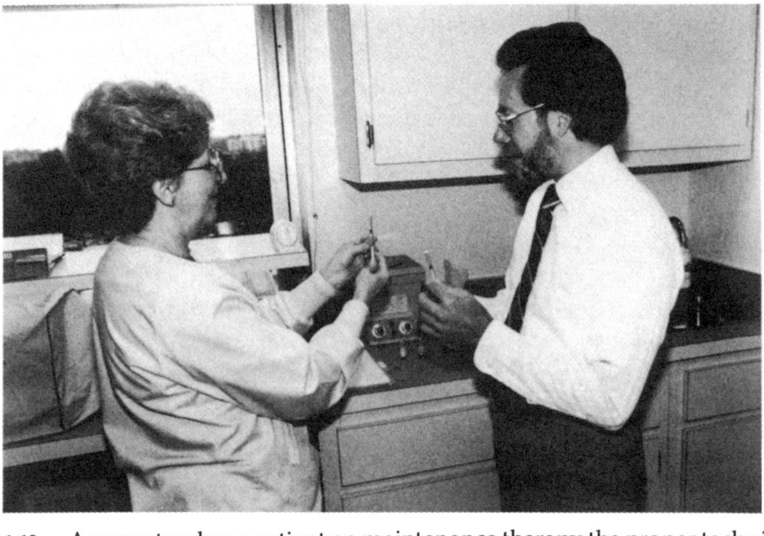

Figure 1-10. A nurse teaches a patient on maintenance therapy the proper technique of reading a syringe and drawing up the correct dose prior to learning how to give his own injection.

Table 1–1. 1993 Most Commonly Used CPT Codes in Otolaryngic Allergy*

95020–95023—	DELETED
95024—	Intradermal tests with allergenic extracts, immediate type reaction, specify number of tests
95027—	SET
**95115—	Professional services for allergen immunotherapy not including allergen extracts; single injection
**95117—	Multiple injections
95120—	Professional services for allergen immunotherapy in prescribing physician's office or institution, including provision of allergenic extract (single antigen)
95125—	Allergy injection of multiple antigens. Specify number of injections.
95135—	Professional services for the supervision of antigens for allergen immunotherapy (Specify number of vials); single antigen, single dose vials
95140—	Multiple antigens, single dose vials
95150—	Professional service for the supervision and provision of antigens for allergen immunotherapy (Specify number of treatments or total volume): single or multiple antigens, one multiple dose vial
95155—	Single or multiple antigens, two or more multiple dose vials
95199—	Unlisted allergy/clinical service or procedure
***99211—	Office or other outpatient visit for the evaluation and management of an established patient that may not require the presence of a physician.
86421—	RAST *in vitro* testing (up to five tests)
86422—	RAST (six or more tests)
86423—	Total IgE

*Additional codes are available for insect venom testing and therapy, spirometry, and other allergy-related procedures. See the current CPT books.
**Commercial Insurance Companies prefer the use of these codes.
***This code is typically used when nurses have conferences with patients regarding diet evaluations, etc.

if testing is coded as "SET" rather than intradermal testing (with the number of individual tests listed).

Time

Time must be allotted to answer patient and staff questions and to discuss patient problems. The more training and experience your assistants have, the more questions they can answer. Some doctors have a special time to answer patient calls; others route calls through the allergy assistant. The allergy assistant must also take the time to question every patient before each injection is given, asking about the response to and any reaction to other previous injection(s). It is also a good time to update the medical history and inquire if the patient has started to take any new medications.

Skin testing should be done only when a physician is in the office. Changes in the "shot hours" must be made 2 to 4 weeks ahead and posted in the office.

OSHA and CLIA

New government regulations have placed stringent requirements on how we practice in our offices—both otolaryngology and allergy. The CLIA regulations require specific quality control techniques and laboratory inspections.

Occupational Safety and Health Administration (OSHA)

OSHA regulations require written policies to be maintained. The easiest method is to use a consulting service which provides all of the forms and labels and itemizes the requirements to put the office in compliance.
To summarize the regulations:

1. Hazard communication policy:
   a. All hazardous chemical substances must be listed and labeled.
   b. Material Safety Data Sheets must be kept on file.
   c. Personnel must be trained in proper cleaning and waste handling.
   d. Fire prevention policies must be outlined.
2. Bloodborne pathogen policy:
   a. An exposure control plan must be written.
   b. Personal protective clothing and equipment must be provided and handwashing rules outlined.
   c. Rules for sharps disposal and infectious waste handling are to be outlined.
   d. Exposure incident report procedure must be in place.
3. An injury and illness prevention program:
   a. Training.
   b. Hazard identification.
   c. Accident investigation.
   d. Documentation and record keeping.

Clinical Laboratory Improvement Act (CLIA)

Documentation is vital. This is the first thing an inspector will check.

1. Test management, including specimen handling, test requisitions, test records, and test reports, must be all documented.
2. Quality control programs—logs must be kept.
   a. Facilities and personnel must meet standards.
   b. Inventory control.
   c. Procedure manual.
   d. Equipment checks.
   e. Quality control records.
3. Proficiency testing.

In vitro allergy testing is considered a test of high complexity and therefore, requires proficiency testing by an approved program with the records being maintained for at least two years.

Registration with CLIA is mandatory. Inspections are done randomly and at a cost to the laboratory.

Conclusion

Take your time getting started. Get organized. Evaluate equipment options but don't buy everything. Examine space needs and economics. Train all personnel well. Order the essentials initially and add additional materials as your allergy practice expands.

· 2 ·

History of Skin Testing and Evolution of Skin Endpoint Titration

JOSEPH P. KEENAN, M.D., F.A.C.S., F.A.A.O.A.

History

Skin testing to determine the degree of allergy in an individual has been used by physicians for the past 100 years. Although early observations that describe allergic reactions in individuals can be found in the writing of Hippocrates, the first modern description of an allergic patient was published by a London physician, Jonathan Bostock, in 1819. In his article "A Case of Periodical Affection of the Eyes and Chest," he clearly described a clinical condition known today as asthma and allergic rhinitis.[1] The term he used to describe this condition was "summer catarrh." He wrote a follow-up paper in 1828 when he further developed his theory of causation for this illness. It was his theory that an effluvium (gas) was produced by the action of sunbeams on freshly mowed hay and it was this effluvium that caused the observed symptoms.

In 1872, Wyman, at Harvard University, clearly identified ragweed pollen as the causative agent in hayfever. This he described in his publication *Autumnal Catarrh*.[2] The following year, Blackley, a physician in Manchester, England, ran a series of experiments in which he performed the first skin test. His protocol consisted of applying grass pollen extract to the excoriated skin of a patient's forearm and demonstrating the development of a wheal in allergic individuals.

In 1911, Leonard Noon, an infectious disease specialist, injected allergic patients with pollen extract in an attempt to cause that patient to develop "pollen antitoxin" to neutralize the "toxin" that he theorized was produced by the body secondary to the original pollen exposure. Leonard Noon also developed a method to standardize the potency of allergic extracts. The protocol he developed involved making various dilutions of an allergic extract that he dropped into the conjunctiva of an allergic individual. The strength of the extract needed to produce erythema and inflammation of the conjunctiva was the endpoint.

As a result of his research, he introduced a definition of allergen potency that is used to this day, namely, the "Noon unit." This unit of measure was originally defined by Noon as "the amount of pollen that could be extracted from the thousandth part of a milligram of Phleum (Timothy) pollen."[3] It should be noted that this definition is based on the arbitrary assumption that 1 g of pollen contained 1 million units. The evolution of this concept today is understood as merely a weight/volume relationship (e.g., weight of pollen in g/ml of extracting fluid). Some approximate equivalencies to keep in mind are:

1 Noon unit = 0.001 mg pollen = 1/2 PNU = 0.1 ml of #4 test solution.

In 1930, French Hansel, an otolaryngologist, began experimenting with skin testing using various dilutions rather than a single test of allergenic material. It was his conclusion that multiple tests using various dilutions of a single antigen gave much more information than using only a single test. This was the natural outgrowth of the observation made earlier by Phillips that the size of the intradermal skin reaction correlated with the antigen dose that could be administered safely to an allergic patient.[4]

In 1937, Rinkel, a general allergist, as a result of his work with Hansel, refined the concept of skin endpoint titration. He carried out many different testing protocols using various dilutions of the antigenic material. It was his observation that the most reliable, reproducible, and clinically helpful information was to be gained using the 1:5 dilution technique. He felt that this technique of skin endpoint titration was superior because both a qualitative and quantitative measure of allergic reactivity was obtained with its use.

Techniques of Testing

Scratch Testing

Scratch testing is the original technique first described by Charles Blackley in 1873. This technique consists of making 2-mm superficial lacerations in the patient's skin followed by the application of a drop of concentrated antigen.

Its advantages are:

1. safe, rarely causes systemic reaction.
2. lack of delayed skin reaction.
3. concentrates that are used are economical and have a long shelf life.

Its disadvantages are:

1. false positive (irritation of skin rather than allergic reaction) results can occur.
2. more painful.
3. not as reproducible as an intradermal skin test.

Because of limited reproducibility and other drawbacks, this form of testing is no longer a recommended diagnostic procedure, according to the Allergy Panel of the AMA Council on Scientific Affairs.[5]

Prick Tests

The technique of the prick test was first described by Lewis and Grant in 1926.[6] As currently performed, a single drop of antigen concentrate is placed on the skin. A sterile 26-gauge needle is passed through this drop and inserted into the skin in a superficial manner so that no bleeding is caused. A variant of this test is the "multitest," in which a sterile disposable applicator with eight puncture heads is used, which allows for the simultaneous testing of six antigens and a positive (histamine) and negative (glycerine) control. Grading of skin reactivity is done on a subjective 0 through 4+ basis.

Its advantages are:

1. rapid screening.
2. better correlation with intradermal tests.
3. relatively safe.

Its disadvantages are:

1. gives qualitative measure of allergy only.
2. will miss low degree of allergy (false negative).
3. grading of skin test is subjective.

The prick test is a rapid way to screen for multiple antigens. If the skin test is positive, then the patient is almost certainly allergic, but the converse is not true. If the patient has a positive history and a negative prick test, the physician is obliged to proceed with intradermal testing.

Intradermal Tests

The first description of the intradermal skin test was made by Robert Cooke in 1915.[7] The technique has undergone few modifications since that time. As described today, the procedure is to use a 26-gauge needle to inject intradermally a small amount of antigen, variously reported to range from 0.01 to 0.05 ml. The concentration of the extract ranges from 1:500 to 1:1000. The tests are read at 10 to 15 minutes. The erythema and whealing are measured and graded on a subjective scale of 0 through 4+.

Its advantages are:

1. highly sensitive (low degree of allergy detected).
2. reproducible.

Its disadvantages are:

1. qualitative but not quantitative.
2. grading of response is subjective.
3. no standardization as to the amount or concentration of test dose.

The intradermal test is a good test, sensitive and highly reproducible. Accuracy is clearly improved by testing with various dilutions of extract but lack of standardization of testing protocol regarding volume and concentration of test dose as well as degree of subjectivity in grading the skin response are serious drawbacks to this original technique.

Skin Endpoint Titration

The development of skin endpoint titration (SET) is a natural outgrowth and refinement of the single dilution intradermal skin test. In fact, a form of SET is used by the Office of Biologic Research and Review (a part of the Food and Drug Administration) to standardize allergic extracts.[8] As previously discussed, the technique of SET was first developed by Hansel and subsequently refined by Rinkel, who introduced the concept of the 1:5 dilution.

The actual technique of SET is described elsewhere in this volume, but a brief description of some of the key concepts is appropriate here. Fivefold dilution of the allergenic extracts are made and these are labeled dilutions #1 through #6. The #1 dilution is five times weaker than the concentrate (1:20 in most cases), so the weight per volume designation of the #1 dilution would be 1:100. The same procedure is followed to make the remaining dilutions.

The test material, starting with the #6 dilution, is injected intradermally. Only 0.01 cc of the extract is used, which will make a 4-mm wheal that enlarges (without reaction) to 5 mm by diffusion. If there is no significant growth of the wheal after 10 minutes, the next stronger dilution (#5) is similarly injected. In the allergic individual, a progression of the whealing response will be observed. The endpoint is defined as that dilution that initiates progressive positive whealing.

Once the endpoint is determined, the individual treatment vials are made, taking into account the quantitative and qualitative aspects of that patient's allergic disease.

Its advantages are:

1. quantitative as well as qualitative measure of allergy.
2. highly reproducible.
3. very sensitive.
4. safe.

Its disadvantages are:

1. time-consuming test procedure.
2. questionable clinical importance at demonstrated low degrees of allergy.
3. more supplies needed (syringes/needles, etc.).

SET has been approved by the Allergy Panel of the AMA Council of Scientific Affairs as being both useful and effective in the diagnosis of allergy.[5] To encourage standardization in use of this procedure, the AAOA has developed a protocol that should be followed closely by physicians using this technique.

References

1. Bostock J. Case of periodical affection of the eyes and chest. *Med Chr Trans* 1819;10:161.
2. Wyman M. *Autumnal Catarrh*. Cambridge: Hurd & Houghton, 1872.
3. Noon L. Prophylactic inoculation for hay fever. *Lancet* 1911;1:1572.
4. Phillips EW. Relief of hayfever by intradermal injections of pollen extract. *JAMA* 1926;86: 182–184.
5. Council on Scientific Affairs (AMA): In vivo diagnostic testing and immunotherapy for allergy. *JAMA* 1987;258:1363–1367.
6. Lewis T, Grant RT. Vascular reactions of the skin to injury. *Heart* 1926;13:219–225.
7. Cooke RA. The treatment of hay fever by active immunization. *Laryngoscope* 1915;25:108–112.
8. Turkeltaub PC, et al. A standardized quantitative skin test assay of allergen potency and stability. *Allergy Clin Immunol* 1982;70:343–352.

· 3 ·

*Whealing Responses**

RICHARD L. MABRY, M.D., F.A.C.S., F.A.A.O.A.

The diagnosis of upper respiratory allergy begins with a thorough and ongoing history. A complete examination of the head and neck, sometimes combined with fiberoptic endoscopy, provides important diagnostic information. Ancillary tests such as a nasal smear and/or sinus radiographs are often helpful. However, the definitive diagnosis of immunoglobulin E (IgE)-mediated nasal and upper respiratory atopy has for years depended on the results of skin testing. Newer modalities for *in vitro* determination of antigen-specific IgE are also helpful, but such tests must be confirmed by some type of skin test, such as a vial test, and skin tests may be necessary for antigens not available for *in vitro* testing. Therefore, it is mandatory that the individual wishing to treat patients with upper respiratory allergy be thoroughly familiar with skin testing—both the theory and the technique.

Whealing Response

Injection of 0.01 ml of any liquid (antigen, diluent, saline) produces a wheal approximately 4 mm in diameter, which soon grows to about 5 mm by physical spreading. Positive responses enlarge beyond this by the production of a "wheal and flare" response. For such a response to occur skin mast cells (of which about 10,000/mm^3 of skin are normally present) must have antigen-

*Adapted with permission from Mabry RL. *SET: History, Theory, and Technique*. Round Rock, TX: Meridian Bio-Medical, 1992.

specific IgE affixed to them. When the specific antigen bridges adjacent IgE units, chemical mediators including histamine are released, producing a Gell and Coombs type I hypersensitivity reaction. The immediate response phase of this reaction produces the wheal and accompanying flare. The wheal begins to grow within 2 to 5 minutes, and enlarges to maximum size at 10 to 15 minutes. (Later wheal enlargement is often due to a Gell and Coombs type III or IV reaction, and has a different significance than the acute reaction. Such a late reaction is most often associated with mold hypersensitivity.) Local vasodilation produces the accompanying flare response, but although erythema should be noted in reading skin tests, only the diameter of the palpable induration at 10 to 15 minutes determines the reaction.

Positive Whealing and Skin Endpoint Titration

If a hypersensitivity ("allergic"). reaction is present, a positive wheal will enlarge at least an additional 2 mm beyond the size of the "negative" (5 mm) wheal within 10 minutes. Rinkel showed that if progressively stronger (five-fold) concentrations of antigen were applied, each succeeding positive wheal would be at least 2 mm larger than the preceding one. He defined the "endpoint" as the dilution that initiates progressive positive whealing; in other words, the first dilution that yields a wheal at least 2 mm larger than the preceding negative wheal and that is followed by a wheal at the next stronger dilution that is at least 2 mm larger still. This second positive wheal is called a "confirming wheal" and is important in defining a true endpoint. This method of determining the level of positive reaction is termed "skin endpoint titration" (Figs. 3-1 and 3-2). Examples (endpoint underlined) are:

5-5-7-9 (if carried further, -11-13, etc.)
5-5-7-7-9 (plateau reaction . . . see below)
5-8-11 (variable increment . . . see below).

Unusual Whealing Responses

It must first be recognized that although the classic description of progressive whealing indicates enlargement by 2-mm increments, the actual size of a positive wheal may be 3 or 4 mm (or more) larger than the preceding one. Thus, a *variant increment whealing response* may be observed with a progression of:

5-5-8-11

The other common normal variant is a *plateau response*, in which two (or more) of the positive wheals are the same size. For example:

5-5-7-7-9

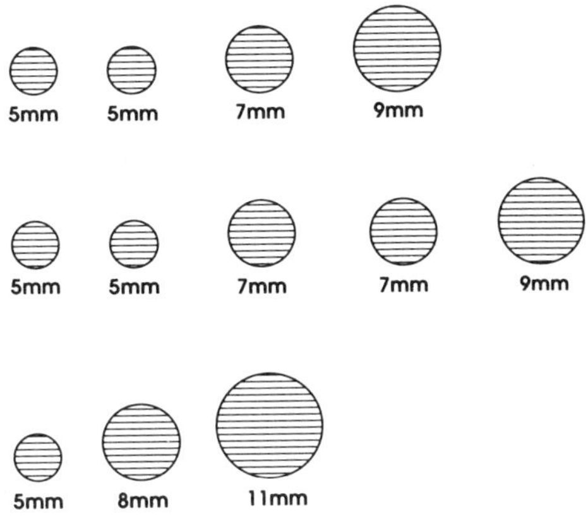

Figure 3-1. Typical whealing response.

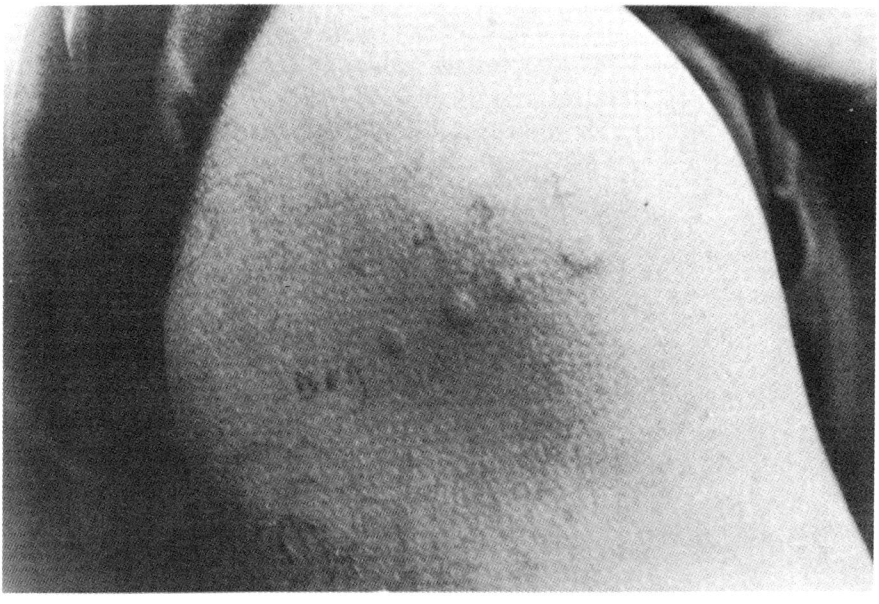

Figure 3-2. A series of uniform wheals of increasing strength have been administered. After 10 minutes, a progressive gradation in size is evident, indicating both the degree of sensitivity to the antigen and a safe strength at which to initiate immunotherapy. (Reprinted from King H. *An Otolaryngologist's Guide to Allergy*. New York: Thieme Medical Publishers, 1990.)

The positive response furthest to the right, followed by the confirming wheal, is normally considered the endpoint, as it initiates *progressive* positive whealing.

An abnormal variant may occur, in which a series of negative responses is suddenly followed by a large positive wheal. For example:

5-5-5-15

Such a response is called a *flash response*, and is usually considered to be due to a concomitant food allergy. When a flash response is obtained, the safest course is to return the patient for retesting the next day, at which time the true endpoint is usually apparent. Confusion may exist in differentiating a flash response from a variant whealing configuration. The former is characterized by negative wheals followed abruptly by a wheal that is much larger (often 10 mm) than the negative wheal. In a variant whealing response, a progression will be seen when the confirming wheal is applied.

Another example of variant whealing is an *hourglass response*. In this, wheals of decreasing size are followed by a clear zone, after which the usual progression appears:

9-7-5-5-$\underline{7}$-9

This "underdose response" is observed most frequently when testing begins at a very dilute level (weaker than #6). Since *in vitro* studies have shown that testing and treatment can be instituted safely at a #6 dilution in the great majority of instances, hourglass reactions are now rarely observed.

Factors Modifying Whealing

The size of the skin reaction is influenced by a number of factors, including the volume and potency of allergen injected, the degree of sensitization of cutaneous mast cells (related to levels of circulating IgE specific for that allergen), and the reactivity of the skin to histamine and other mediators released from the mast cells. The response is also modified by drugs, the presence of blocking antibodies, the age and race of the patient, the area of the body injected, the distance separating individual skin tests, and the time of day of testing.

A wheal's initial size is directly related to the volume injected. For example, 0.01 ml is said to produce a wheal of about 4 mm, which enlarges to about 5 mm due to physical spreading. If the volume injected is increased to about 0.05 ml, the resulting wheal is about 7 to 9 mm.

The reactivity of the sensitized skin mast cells and the degree of antigenicity of the solution injected affect the amount of histamine and other vasoactive amines liberated as a result of a skin test, and thus affect the size of the ultimate wheal. The skin of some individuals is overly responsive to trauma, and a wheal and flare response will be seen in these patients (who are dermatographic) even after the injection of an inert substance. For this reason, a negative control is always necessary when skin testing (see below).

Allergen exposure has the same effect on skin reactivity as the use of stronger testing antigen; that is, the production of a more intense skin reaction. Therefore, patients will usually be found to be more sensitive to skin testing carried out during the season when the allergens are at their peak, and endpoints obtained during coseasonal testing will often shift when that antigen goes out of season.

Antihistamines suppress the wheal and flare response. With almost all common antihistamines, this effect has effectively ceased within 24 hours or less of the delivery of the last medication to the body and skin testing may thus be carried out if the patient has taken no such drugs for 36 hours. Short-acting antihistamines such as diphenhydramine and triprolidine can often be given the day before testing without affecting skin responses. However, astemizole has an extremely slow clearance rate for the drug and its metabolites from the body, and if tissue saturation has been obtained by prolonged therapy, at least 3 weeks must elapse after cessation of astemizole therapy before skin testing is carried out (with a histamine control applied to evaluate the integrity of the wheal and flare response).

Bear in mind that antihistamines are also contained in or include some soporifics, cough syrups, "cold" remedies, antipruritics, and anxiolytics.

Tricyclic antidepressants have been observed to suppress skin test responses for from 2 to 4 days after administration of these compounds.

Decongestants, cromolyn, corticosteroids, and bronchodilators do not affect skin test results, and need not be discontinued before testing.

Patients who have undergone previous treatment may have altered skin test responses as compared to pretreatment levels, due to the production of IgG4-blocking antibodies, as well as from a lowered level of allergen-specific IgE.

The skin of some patients, especially infants and the elderly, is said to be less reactive to skin testing than that of the population as a whole. A general decline of skin reactivity after the age of 50 has been described, although specific IgE measurement by *in vitro* means has shown that allergy continues to exist in this age group. The area of the body skin tested affects the size of the resultant wheals. Decreasing reactivity of skin is found in the mid and upper back > lower back > upper arm > elbow > forearm (ulnar > radial) > wrist. Finally, the skin is said to be up to 2½ times more responsive to tests applied between 7:00 and 11:00 PM as compared to those applied at 7:00 AM.

Axonal reflexes may affect the results of skin tests. Positive skin tests or histamine controls placed too near other skin tests can initiate axonal reflexes that drive the wheal and flare response. Thus, the histamine control should be placed well away from other tests, and individual skin tests should be separated by at least 2 cm. (Some authorities advise a 5-cm separation, which is laudable but impractical in most instances.)

Concomitant foods are foods that react along with inhalants to enhance both symptom production and skin reactivity. Classic examples include watermelon (and other members of the gourd family) with ragweed, birch with apple, grass with cereal grains, and so forth. Ingestion of a concomitant food before testing with a related inhalant antigen will usually result in a flash response (described above), or in an endpoint falsely shifted to the left (endpoint at a more dilute antigen strength).

Controls To Assess Skin Reactivity

1. *Diluent*: A 4-mm wheal of diluent (phenolated saline) should give a wheal of about 5 mm after 10 minutes. If a wheal of 7 mm or more results from this injection, the patient is probably dermatographic, and skin testing may have to be abandoned in favor of *in vitro* methods.

2. *Histamine control*: For years, histamine phosphate in a concentration of 2.75 mg/5 ml was used as a stock solution to prepare serial five-fold dilutions, and the #3 dilution of this material was applied as a positive skin test control. Since this stock concentration of histamine is no longer readily available, it may be necessary to use histamine phosphate in a concentration of 0.275 mg/ml as a beginning point. Using this stock solution, the #3 histamine control is prepared as follows:

Withdraw and discard 1 ml from a sterile vial that contains 4 ml of sterile diluent. To the remaining 3 ml, add 2 ml of histamine phosphate, 0.275 mg/ml. The mixture resulting is equivalent to the #1 dilution of histamine prepared using the stronger stock material. Add 1 ml of this #1 strength to 4 ml of sterile diluent, to prepare a #2 histamine dilution. One more five-fold dilution is necessary to prepare a #3 concentration.

When applied as an intradermal skin test to create a 5 mm wheal, histamine #3 should produce a wheal which enlarges to at least 7 mm in diameter within 10 minutes. Such a reaction confirms the integrity of the wheal and flare capability of the skin. If the histamine control is non-reactive (not enlarging at least 2 mm or more), skin testing at this time will not be accurate, and a search must be made for medications or other factors rendering the skin hyposensitive.

3. *Glycerine #2*: Fifty percent glycerine diluted twice in the usual 1:5 fashion to a #2 dilution (using the 50% concentration as concentrate) yields a solution containing 2% glycerine. Antigen concentrates contain 50% glycerine as a preservative, so a #2 dilution of a concentrate contains 2% glycerine. This usually gives a wheal of 5 to 7 mm. Therefore, if a 7-mm or larger wheal results with glycerine #2, a positive response to any #2 test dilution may be due to the glycerine, not the antigen, and one must exercise clinical judgment as to its significance.

If testing with an antigen at a #1 dilution, a comparable wheal of #1 glycerine must be applied, and the wheal sizes compared in order to assess the significance of the results.

Suggested Readings

Galant SP, et al. The inhibitory effect of antiallergy drugs on allergen and histamine induced wheal and flare response. *J Allergy Clin Immunol* 1973;51:11–21.
King WP. The role of skin endpoint titration method in allergy. In Goldman JL, ed. *The Principles and Practice of Rhinology*, pp 283–292, New York, John Wiley & Sons, 1987.
Long WF, et al. Skin test suppression by antihistamines and the development of subsensitivity. *J Allergy Clin Immunol* 1985;76:113–117.
Nelson HS. Diagnostic procedures in allergy. I. Allergy skin testing. *Ann Allergy* 1983;51:411.
Rao SK, et al. Duration of the suppressive effect of tricyclic antidepressants on histamine induced wheal-and-flare reaction in human skin. *J Allergy Clin Immunol* 1988;82:752–757.
Rinkel HJ. The management of clinical allergy (1, 11, 111). *Arch Otolaryngol* 1962;76:491–508, 1963;77:42–75, 1963;77: 205–235.

· 4 ·

Antigen Choice for Testing

WILLIAM P. KING, M.D., F.A.C.S., F.A.A.O.A.

Biologic inhalant antigens may be classified as pollens, molds, and household perennials. The selection of appropriate antigens for testing and treatment is of great importance to the physician beginning an allergy practice. The discussion that follows addresses this problem.

Pollens

In choosing pollens for testing and treatment, one must consider Thommen's postulates.[1] These state that, to be allergenically significant, the following characteristics are necessary:

1. The plant must be seed-bearing, with pollen wind-borne (*anemophilous*), for wide distribution. (This removes from consideration plants with showy flowers and sticky pollen, which are typically insect pollinated.)
2. The pollen must be produced in large quantities.
3. The pollen must be buoyant, in order to be distributed over a wide area. (Pollen from 15 to 50 μm in diameter meet this test.)
4. The plant must be widely and abundantly distributed, preferably close to human habitation.
5. The pollen must be allergenic. (That is, it must be capable of producing an allergic reaction, rather than mere irritation.)

The first consideration in choosing pollen antigens is the list of most common plants in the area (which meet criteria 1–4 above). A "must" source for such an evaluation is Lewis' text, *Airborne and Allergenic Pollen of North America*,[2] which provides comprehensive information about plant distribution. Further details of indigenous plants may be obtained from local libraries, agricultural and gardening authorities, schools and colleges, and so forth. Armed with this information, a first-hand survey of potential local offending plants should be carried out. Antigen distributors may also provide information regarding plant distribution and pollen seasons, plus information gained from their experience in providing for the needs of other physicians in the area. If available, specific pollen counts provide precise information about the variety, prevalence, and persistence of specific pollens. Ideally, these should be accomplished at least weekly over 1 to 3 years to minimize variability. If the physician is not able to perform his own pollen counts, local health departments sometimes provide this information.

Once having chosen pollens (and other antigens) for testing and treatment, the selections will be modified over time by experience with patients. For instance, one general rule is to purchase initially the smallest amount possible of each antigen. If the vial has not been emptied before its expiration date is reached (i.e., not enough patients have been placed on treatment with the antigen to use it up), serious consideration should be given to its removal from your board.

A great consideration in choosing pollens is cross-reactivity. This phenomenon exists when the specific antibody produced in response to one allergen also reacts with one or more other (similar) allergens. Cross-reactivity, although suspected in the past, has been extensively investigated more recently by radioallergosorbent test (RAST) inhibition studies. It is important to realize that including a number of cross-reacting antigens in a treatment set can result in significant local or systemic reactions because of effective overdosing.

Cross-reactivity is of greater significance in the case of pollens than molds or household perennials. The most thorough documentation of this phenomenon involves grasses. Five families of grasses are recognized. The most significant are the Pooideae (most familiar lawn and wild grasses, including brome, fescue, june/blue, orchard, perennial rye, quack, redtop, sweet vernal, timothy, velvet, and western wheat) and the Chloridoideae (mainly bermuda and grama grass). Strong cross-reactivity exists within the Pooideae, and perennial rye or timothy are typically chosen for testing and treating this entire family, as either contains all or almost all epitopes. The Chloridoideae show only minor epitope-sharing with the Pooideae; Bermuda (which contains all the epitopes for this family) is the prototype for testing in this family.

Members of the third grass family, the Panicoideae (bahia, Johnson grass, sorghum, crabgrass), have many epitopes in common with the first two families mentioned. Bahia has the fewest common epitopes, and when prominent in an area, should be tested and treated separately. Johnson grass, if locally present in large amounts, is handled similarly.

The last two grass families contain reeds, rice and wild rice, and bamboo, and are usually not included in treatment sets unless local circumstances warrant.

In a fashion similar to grasses, weeds are known to cross-react. The largest family of weeds is the Composites (family Asteraceae) composed of three tribes, the Astereae (goldenrod, Baccharis species), the Anthemideae (mugwort, sage, sagebrush, wormwood), and the Heliantheae (marsh elder, cocklebur, ragweed varieties). Although unproven, suspicion of reasonable cross-sensitivity in the first two groups may allow testing of only the most locally prominent member. The members of the Helianths are generally not felt to cross-react significantly except for the ragweed varieties (short, giant, Western). All of these cross-react, allowing testing for only one member. The most commonly used is short ragweed.

The other major weed group is the Cheno-Ams, composed of the Chenopod family (Russian thistle, burning bush, lamb's quarters, Atriplex) and the Amaranth family (pigweed, careless weed, tumbleweed). Although some cross-reactivity is suspected, they are generally tested for separately. The exceptions are members of the Triplex genus (saltbush, shadscale, spearscale, wingscale), all of which cross-react, requiring only one representative for testing and treatment.

Trees may be classified as angiosperms (flowering trees) and gymnosperms (cypress family). Although limited cross-reactivity within the gymnosperms and among closely related angiosperms has been suggested, trees should be tested individually depending on local prevalence.

Despite not fulfilling some other criteria, a specific pollen may deserve inclusion in a test battery for specific patients. Examples are cottonwood (not usually considered highly allergenic) in the patient whose house is situated in a cottonwood grove. Likewise, although pine pollen is not widely airborne, the individual whose occupation places him beneath pine trees for extended periods may deserve testing for the antigen.

A typical full pollen battery includes no more than two to three grasses, five to seven weeds, and four to seven trees.

Molds

Mold growth is most prevalent in warmer areas with high humidity. Seasonal variation depends on climate. Generally speaking, mold spores are an important allergenic consideration east of the Mississippi River. In the drier western regions, molds are said to be less common but may still be significant in the total allergic picture. Further, realize that outside airborne mold spore counts are not indicative of the individual's home and workplace indoor mold exposure. In the home, mold growth is commonly seen on bathroom tile, on indoor plants, and so forth. Furthermore, the use of mold mixes is not recommended. (Indeed, the AAOA does not advocate the use of any mixes, except in the case of certain closely related antigens such as white-red-Virginia oak or giant-short-western ragweed.)

Recent studies using RAST testing for mold allergies have emphasized the significance of the many varieties of mold. Past experiences have indicated that Alternaria is the most prevalent and allergenic of the common molds, followed closely by Helminthosporium and Cladosporium (depending on geographic location). Some other common airborne offenders currently available for specific testing and treatment include Curvularia, Epicoccum, Fusarium, Stemphylium, Aspergillus, Mucor, Penicillium, Aureobasidium, Botrytis, Phoma, and Rhizopus. Thus, air sampling becomes very important to assess the local airborne mold population. When indoor molds are problematic, the use of mold plates may be necessary for adequate evaluation.

Depending on the area, approximately 10 molds may be advised for testing in a complete battery.

Household Perennials

The category of household perennials contains allergens found year-round in the house. Most prominent within this group is the house dust mite. Other household perennial allergens are cockroach, animal danders (pets or livestock), and feathers (from birds or stuffing). A study in which 100 patients were tested for inhalants by a full battery of RAST antigens indicated that if only one or two positive reactors were found, these were usually household perennials. These may be the only positive allergens in a test battery, but can produce severe symptoms. All such perennials to which a patient is exposed should be included in the original test battery.

Like mold, house dust mite is most often noted in humid, low-lying areas. A study by Scadding and Brostoff[3] showed that in London the housedust mite population varied inversely with the distance of the house from the Thames River. Dust mite allergy at high altitudes, such as in Denver, is not usually a significant problem.

Four major species of house dust mite are recognized: *Dermatophagoides farinae*, *D pteronyssinus*, *D microceras*, and *Euroglyphus maynei*. Only the first two, which represent the more common species found in the United States, are available for testing and treatment. Because of strongly shared epitopes, testing and treatment for *D farinae* suffices, although in some instances adding *D pteronyssinus* yields superior patient responses. Both these species weakly cross-react with *D microceras*.

Cockroach is a major allergenic offender in certain areas. Additionally, testing for all danders and pet-related allergens to which the patient is exposed (depending on a thorough history) should be carried out.

In some locations, kissing bugs may present an allergenic problem. The local species must be identified to obtain optimum response from testing and treatment if an antigen for this insect can be obtained.

Screens

It is neither necessary nor advisable to perform initially a full battery of inhalant tests. Screening techniques have been demonstrated to be effective, whether testing is performed by skin tests or *in vitro* means. A 1982 study by King[4] and a 1985 study by Nalebuff[5] showed the efficacy of using a "screening" RAST panel. The first study showed that approximately one-third of initial full test batteries were negative, and one-sixth were positive only for household perennials. In King's studies, the efficiency and sensitivity of a screen was shown to be in the neighborhood of 95%. Initially, King proposed a screen comprising three pollens (the most prevalent area grass, weed, and tree), two molds (Alternaria and Cladosporium), and all household perennials deemed appropriate according to individual exposure. In 1989, an additional study by King[6] advised adding Helminthosporium to the mold panel for most areas. (The reader is referred to the articles cited for full details of the studies.)

Example of Screening Panel (South Texas)

Grass:	Rye
Weed:	Short ragweed
Tree:	Oak
Molds:	Alternaria
	Cladosporium
	Helminthosporium
Household perennials:	*D. farinae*
	Cockroach
	Animal danders (as indicated by history)

The specific antigens used for screening will obviously vary from area to area, differing primarily in the pollens chosen (less so for molds and household perennials). If the screening test is negative (as was the case in one-third of the tests in King's study cited above) inhalant testing is ended. The same is true if only household perennials are positive. If pollens or molds are positive, all remaining antigens in that category must be tested.

Conclusion

Presented for your review is a system for choosing an armamentarium of inhalant allergens for testing in a specific geographic area. A full test battery may include up to 17 pollens, 10 molds, and three or more household perennials (a total of 30 or more antigens). However, 8 to 12 appropriate antigens used as a screen may be sufficient, in up to half the patients tested, to rule out significant inhalant allergy or define household perennials as the only positive allergen, avoiding both unnecessary testing and expense.

References

1. Coca A, Thommen AS, Walzer A. *Asthma and Hayfever Plants in Theory and in Practice.* Springfield, IL: Charles C Thomas, 1931.
2. Lewis WH, Vinary P, Zenger VE. *Airborne and Allergenic Pollen of North America.* Baltimore: Johns Hopkins University Press, 1983.
3. Scadding G, Brostoff J. Low dose sublingual therapy in patients with allergic rhinitis due to house dust mite. *Clin Allergy* 1986;16:483–491.
4. King WP. Efficacy of a screening radioallergosorbent test. *Arch Otolaryngol* 1982;108:781–786.
5. Nalebuff DJ. Use of RAST screening in clinical allergy: A cost effective approach to patient care. *Ear Nose Throat J* 1985;64:15–35.
6. King WP. Clinical significance of molds newly available for RAST testing. *Otolaryngol Head Neck Surg* 1989;101:1–4.

· 5 ·

Technique of Skin Endpoint Titration

HAMILTON S. DIXON, M.D., F.A.A.O.A.
B. JANE DIXON, B.S., F.A.A.O.A.

Instructions for Mixing Test Sets

1. Arrange and label 5-cc bottles for each allergen to be included in the testing set. The bottles contain 4 cc of diluent. Example: first group—Ragweed. Label six bottles Ragweed, nos. 1 through 6, and the date. Do this for all allergens to be included in the testing set.

2. Refer to Table 5-1, "Mixing Test or Treatment Sets" (p. 36). There are two columns, one for 1:20 concentrates and one for 1:10 concentrates.

3. The left-hand column instructions are for mixing most pollen allergens, which are 1:20 concentrates.

To make dilution #1, use a 5-cc vial with 4.0 cc of premeasured diluent. To that 4.0 cc of diluent add 1.0 cc of the allergen concentrate. This gives a total volume of 5.0 cc in bottle #1 (1:100).

With bottle #2 ready, withdraw 1.0 cc from bottle #1. Inject this 1.0 cc into bottle #2 and rinse syringe five to six times. With bottle #3 ready, withdraw 1.0 cc from bottle #2 and inject into bottle #3. Continue with the same method to as high a dilution as you wish to mix (in most cases, a #6 dilution). The same syringe may be used for one allergen with successively weaker dilutions only if the plunger is pushed in and out five to six times (rinsing).

4. The right-hand column instructions are for mixing some inhalant aller-

gens (dust and molds), foods, and special mixtures that usually come as 1:10 concentrates.

Begin with a 4.0-cc bottle of premeasured diluent. To this *add an additional 0.50 cc of diluent* from a separate bottle (usually from a 100-cc bottle included in your supply list). The #1 bottle now has 4.5 cc of diluent. To this #1 bottle add 0.50 cc of allergen concentrate. We now have a total volume of 5.0 cc of the #1 mixture (1:100).

With bottle #2 ready, withdraw 1.0 cc from bottle #1 and inject into bottle #2, rinsing the syringe five to six times. Repeat this procedure all the way up to bottle #6 or as high as you wish to mix.

5. An important point to remember: the stability of the allergen is directly related to the amount of its dilution. The testing set is valid up to 2 months, but within the 2-month period, the #1 dilution is obviously more stable than #2 through #6, due to its glycerine content. (Phenolated saline diluent is good for 6–8 weeks, if refrigerated when not in use.)

Controls

Before skin testing is begun, positive and negative controls should be done.

Histamine Control

For years, histamine phosphate in a concentration of 2.75 mg/5 ml was used as a stock solution to prepare serial five-fold dilutions, and the #3 dilution of this material was applied as a positive skin test control. Since this stock concentration of histamine is no longer readily available, it may be necessary to use histamine phosphate in a concentration of 0.275 mg/ml as a beginning point. Using this stock solution, the #3 histamine control is prepared as follows:

Withdraw and discard 1 ml from a sterile vial which contains 4 ml of sterile diluent. To the remaining 3 ml, add 2 ml of histamine phosphate, 0.275 mg/ml. The mixture resulting is equivalent to the #1 dilution of histamine prepared using the stronger stock material. Add 1 ml of this #1 strength to 4 ml of sterile diluent, to prepare a #2 histamine dilution. One more five-fold dilution is necessary to prepare a #3 concentration.

When applied as an intradermal skin test to create a 5 mm wheal, histamine #3 should produce a wheal which enlarges to at least 7 mm in diameter within 10 minutes. Such a reaction confirms the integrity of the wheal and flare capability of the skin. If the histamine control is non-reactive (not enlarging at least 2 mm or more), skin testing at this time will not be accurate, and a search must be made for medications or other factors rendering the skin hyposensitive.*

*From Mabry RL. *Skin Endpoint Titration: History, Theory, and Practice (3rd Ed)*. Round Rock, TX: Hycor Biomedical, 1993. Reprinted with permission.

Glycerine Control

1. Start with 50% glycerine as the concentrate and make 1:5 dilutions up to #3.
2. Apply tests with all applicable dilutions by injecting a 4-mm wheal for each. The #1 dilution = 10% glycerine, #2 = 2%, and #3 = 0.4%.
3. Measure wheal size in 10 minutes.
4. Since allergen concentrates come mixed in 50% glycerine from the manufacturer in order to maintain potency and stability, one must be certain that a positive skin test is caused by a hypersensitivity reaction to the allergen, not the glycerine. Thus, it is necessary to compare test wheals at #1, #2, and sometimes #3 dilutions with comparable strengths of glycerine alone. A truly positive reaction should consist of a wheal at least 2 mm larger than the glycerine control for that dilution.

Negative Control

A 4-mm wheal of diluent alone should be applied and should enlarge to no more than 5 or 6 mm at 10 minutes. A larger ("positive") wheal indicates skin hyperactivity (i.e., dermatographia), and skin testing may not be valid in this patient.

Skin Endpoint Titration Mechanics

The outside of the patient's upper arm is used to do skin endpoint titration (SET).

1. Thoroughly cleanse both upper arms with alcohol and dry with a clean dry gauze sponge.
2. Prepare the arm by initialing with the first letter or a symbol for each allergen to be tested, horizontally across the top of the test area. Down the side of the arm, write the numbers 6, 5, 4, 3, 2, 1 vertically. These are the dilutions to be tested. Allow at least a 1" area for each allergen to be tested.
3. From the test rack, remove all necessary dilution #6 bottles (1:312,500) and place them within reach.
4. Using a 27-gauge, ½" bevel needle, withdraw about 0.05 cc of the first allergen from the vial into the testing syringe (exact amount is not important).
5. Look at the syringe and turn the bevel of the needle toward you. (Some prefer testing with the bevel down). With the skin of the upper arm held taut with your other hand by grasping it from behind, slowly inject a sufficient amount of the appropriate allergen (approximately 0.01 ml) intradermally to form a wheal 4 mm in diameter. It is essential to be sure the wheal is raised, indicating a true intradermal placement of the needle. If the needle goes a bit too deep, the wheal will raise poorly and be difficult to measure, thus causing inconsistent results.

6. Proceed with the remaining allergens to be tested at that dilution.
7. When all 4-mm wheals have been applied for the #6 dilution, set the timer for 10 minutes.
8. When the 10-minute timer rings, measure each individual wheal and record the results on the test sheet.
9. Proceed to the next stronger dilution, the #5 (1;62,500), and proceed with test in the same manner.
10. Complete the test by continuing to the #1 dilution or until the endpoint of reaction is established.
11. A second reading of wheals should be done after a total elapsed time of 15 minutes. If any of the wheals have grown further, the larger size should be recorded.

Interpretation of Results

The diagnosis of positive allergens by SET depends on identifying what is called the "endpoint." This is the dilution of an allergen that causes a positive response (at least 2 mm larger than the preceding negative wheal) and is followed by progressive whealing; that is, a 2-mm growth on the next stronger dilution. This endpoint dilution is actually the "starting point" of immunotherapy. It is the dilution used for the initial treatment mixture of each positive antigen.

The interpretation of the whealing response can be valid only if the wheals are injected accurately. The 4-mm wheal must be sharp with well demarcated edges.

When beginning a skin test, one wishes to produce a nonreacting or negative response. The injection of that 4-mm wheal on the #6 dilution should produce a wheal that grows at 10 minutes to no more than 5 or 6 mm in diameter (a negative wheal). If the next stronger dilution produces a wheal at least 2 mm larger, a positive response has been found, but is not necessarily the endpoint. Therefore, do not stop at that point. A wheal with another 2 mm of growth should be found on application of the next stronger dilution to indicate progressive positive whealing and confirm the endpoint.

Testing is stopped when the second progressively reacting wheal is reached. In the examples below, the dilution with the 7-mm wheal immediately preceding the 9-mm wheal represents the endpoint of reaction. A typical test could appear as follows:

# dilutions	#6	#5	#4	#3	#2	#1	EP
Wheal size in mm:	4	4	5	7	9		3 (1:2500)
	5	5	7	9			4 (1:12,500)
	5	7	9				5 (1:62,500)

Table 5–1. Mixing Test or Treatment Sets

1:20 concentrate—pollen allergens
1:10 concentrate—inhalant allergens, foods, special mixtures

	1:20 concentrate	**1:10 concentrate**
Dilution #1	4.00 cc diluent	4.00 cc diluent
		0.50 cc additional diluent
	1.00 cc allergen concentrate	0.50 cc allergen concentrate
Total	5.00 cc	5.00 cc
From this point on, mix both identically		
Dilution #2	4.00 cc diluent	4.00 cc diluent
	1.00 cc #1 allergen	1.00 cc #1 allergen
Total	5.00 cc	5.00 cc
Dilution #3	4.00 cc diluent	4.00 cc diluent
	1.00 cc #2 allergen	1.00 cc #2 allergen
Total	5.00 cc	5.00 cc
Dilution #4	4.00 cc diluent	4.00 cc diluent
	1.00 cc #3 allergen	1.00 cc #3 allergen
Total	5.00 cc	5.00 cc
Dilution #5	4.00 cc diluent	4.00 cc diluent
	1.00 cc #4 allergen	1.00 cc #4 allergen
Total	5.00 cc	5.00 cc

It is not recommended that one apply stronger dilutions to obtain 11- and 13-mm wheals, since this could provoke symptoms and cause patient discomfort. Thus, one stops when progressive whealing is confirmed.

This can be carried out as far as the #6 dilution or higher if needed.

For testing, phenolated saline or albumin saline may be used as the diluent. The dilutions should be mixed to at least the #6 dilution, but up to #10 may be necessary in some instances.

The stability of the allergen is directly related to the amount of its dilution. The testing set is valid up to 2 months if properly mixed and kept refrigerated.

Suggested Readings

King, HC. Endpoint titration and immunotherapy, in Lee KJ (ed), *Otolaryngol Clin No Amer* 18:703–717. Philadelphia: W. B. Saunders, 1985.

King, HC. *An Otolaryngologist's Guide to Allergy*, pp 70–84. New York: Thieme, 1990.

King, WP. The role of skin endpoint titration method in allergy, in Goldman, JL (ed), *The Principles and Practice of Rhinology*, pp 283–292. New York: John Wiley & Sons, 1987.

Mabry RL. *Skin Endpoint Titration: History, Theory, and Practice* (3rd Ed). Round Rock, TX: Hycor Biomedical, 1993.

Rinkel, HJ. The management of clinical allergy, part II, etiologic factors and skin titration. *Arch Otolaryngol* 77:42–75, 1963.

Ward, WA Jr. Diagnostic skin testing: skin endpoint titration, in Krause, HF (ed), *Otolaryngic Allergy and Immunology*, pp. 133–140. Philadelphia: W. B. Saunders, 1989.

· 6 ·

Vial Preparation Based on Skin Endpoint Titration Results

HUESTON C. KING, M.D., F.A.C.S., F.A.A.O.A.

The patient has been diagnosed as atopic (sensitive to airborne allergens) by history, physical examination, and confirmatory skin endpoint titration (SET). The task now remains for preparing the appropriate antigens in a form suitable for the administration of immunotherapy.

A safe starting point for immunotherapy is established by SET. The determination of an endpoint requires the production of a positive wheal (2 mm larger than the preceding negative wheal) and a confirming wheal (a wheal yet 2 mm or more larger after the application of the next stronger dilution). Therefore the test will have administered the antigenic equivalent of .06 cc of the endpoint dilution (0.01 cc of the endpoint, then 0.01 cc of a dilution five times stronger) plus the content of the preceding negative wheal(s). It follows that treatment may safely be begun with 0.05 cc of the endpoint strength.

In the original writings of Rinkel, 0.05 cc of the endpoint dilution was referred to as a "5x dose," and other multiples of this strength could be referred to as 10x (0.10 cc), 50x (0.50 cc), and so forth. Although more concise, this terminology has proved confusing, and will not be used in this manual. However, because of its historical significance, the otolaryngic allergist should be aware of its meaning.

For the patient sensitive to a single antigen, a satisfactory approach might be treating directly from the testing or treatment board with progressively stronger doses from the appropriate vials. However, few patients are sensitive to a single antigen, and administering a separate injection for each antigen is understandably not acceptable to the patient. A means must therefore be found to administer a single injection containing a number of antigens, each at a strength determined by the skin reaction to be both safe and potent, and capable of being escalated without frequent reconstitution. This is done by preparing multidose, multiantigen vials. Reducing the number of separate vials and/or injections, reducing the volume of each injection, and reducing the need for preparing new vials results in both increased safety and patient acceptance.

The calculations necessary for the construction of treatment vials are simple if the principles of the titration format are kept in mind. SET is based on a fivefold serial dilution of antigens. When the amount of antigen used in treatment reaches a volume fivefold greater than that of the original starting dose, the same amount of antigen being used in treatment at that level may be administered by using one fifth of the volume of the next stronger antigen dilution. This reduces by a factor of five the injection volume needed to give the patient the same dose of antigen. The original starting dose for immunotherapy is .05 cc. The maximum dose of a single antigen should be .50 cc, as above this dose conversion to a stronger dilution is indicated.

It is not efficient to make each immunotherapy dose individually. For convenience, it is most efficient to project a multi-dose vial containing 10 doses of .50 cc of each antigen. (The dose immediately in use before converting the vial to the next stronger dilution.) It is not likely that the entire vial will be used before preparing a vial of the next stronger dilution, but the safety and convenience will more than justify the small waste of antigen. To complete the calculations needed for efficiency and simplicity, a 5 cc treatment vial should be prepared. This will contain 10 doses of .50 cc of each antigen to be used in a maximum dose from this vial. Lower doses will be used in an incremental fashion from the vial in escalating treatment. When the .50 cc dose has been reached, the remains of the vial may be discarded in favor of a new vial five times stronger.

In summary, for vial preparation, it is helpful to use antigens in a concentrated form and then add sufficient diluent to yield the desired volume. A number of serial dilutions are necessary for testing, as the amount of each injection must be uniform while the antigenic content increases fivefold with each successively stronger dilution. In therapy, however, the diluent present only adds to the volume of injection. Reduction of diluent may be accomplished by using a smaller amount of a more concentrated strength (still antigenically equivalent) converting to stronger levels up to the limits of reliable measurement. Attempts to measure amounts smaller than 0.1 cc are prone to error.

To prepare a treatment vial containing up to 10 0.5-cc doses, the calculations are as follows:

- maximum dose from treatment vial before converting to a stronger vial = 0.5 cc.
- number of doses = 10, multiplied by 0.5 cc = 5.0 cc total volume of vial

- to remove diluent from a single dose:
  0.5 cc endpoint dilution = 0.1 cc next stronger dilution = 0.02 cc two dilutions stronger.
- to prepare ten such doses:
  0.02 cc two dilutions stronger × 10 = 0.2 cc two dilutions stronger than endpoint dilution.
- to prepare multiple antigen vial, add 0.2 cc two dilutions stronger than endpoint for each positive antigen.
- add diluent to bring total vial content to 5 cc. A dose of 0.5 cc from this vial will contain the antigenic equivalent of 0.5 cc of the endpoint dilution for each antigen in the mix.

Example:

Pollen A	Endpoint #6	0.02 ml of #4 × 10 =	0.20 ml of #4
Pollen B	Endpoint #3	0.02 ml of #1 × 10 =	0.20 ml of #1
Pollen C	Endpoint #5	0.02 ml of #3 × 10 =	0.20 ml of #3
Pollen D	Endpont #4	0.02 ml of #2 × 10 =	0.20 ml of #2
Total antigen			0.80 ml
Diluent added			4.20 ml
Total volume of treatment vial			5.00 ml

Graphic examples of the concentration of an antigen dose: 0.01 cc cannot be measured in the syringe, but produces a 4-mm wheal in the skin; 0.05 cc represents a usual starting dose for immunotherapy, and contains five of the "units" represented by 0.01 cc of antigen; 0.5 cc (Fig. 6-1a) contains 50 of these units, and at this level the dose will have reached the strength of the next stronger dilution. If diluent only is removed from this dose, an amount containing only ⅕ the total volume but the same amount of antigen (50 "units") will result. This is the same as 0.1 cc of the next stronger concentration (Fig. 6-1b). If the same procedure is repeated, the same 50 "units" will be contained in 0.02 cc of the strength two dilutions stronger than the endpoint (Fig. 6-1c). Diluent has been removed by reversing the titration preparation process, but the amount of antigen present has been preserved.

Multiple antigens are delivered from a multiple dose vial at the same rate as are individual antigens. .05 cc of a single-antigen vial delivers 5 .01 "units" of the single antigen. .05 cc of a multiple-antigen vial gives 5 "units" of each antigen.

When the 0.5-cc dosage level is reached, a new vial may be made with each antigen one concentration stronger, and dosage escalation continued. A dose of 0.1 cc of the new vial will have the antigenic equivalence of 0.5 cc from the preceding (fivefold weaker) treatment vial.

The figures given are for a 5-cc vial. If smaller amounts are desired, a 2.5-cc vial may be made by dividing all of the amounts by 2 (i.e., 0.1 cc of antigens, with diluent to make 2.5 cc total), and so on for any size vial the physician wishes to use for maximum convenience and cost effectiveness.

It should be noted that stock antigens are normally purchased in 50%

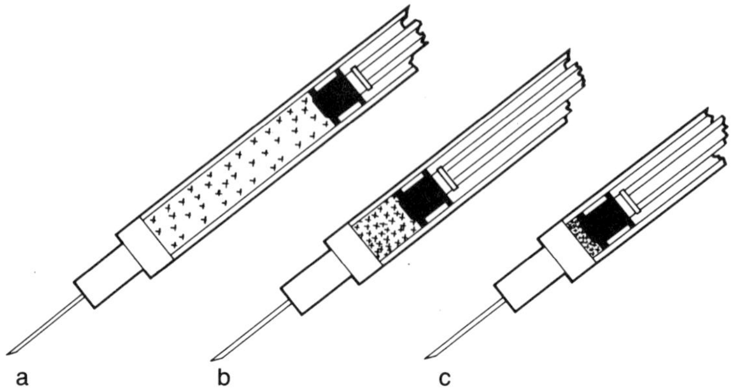

Figure 6-1. **a–c**: Examples of the concentration of an antigen dose.

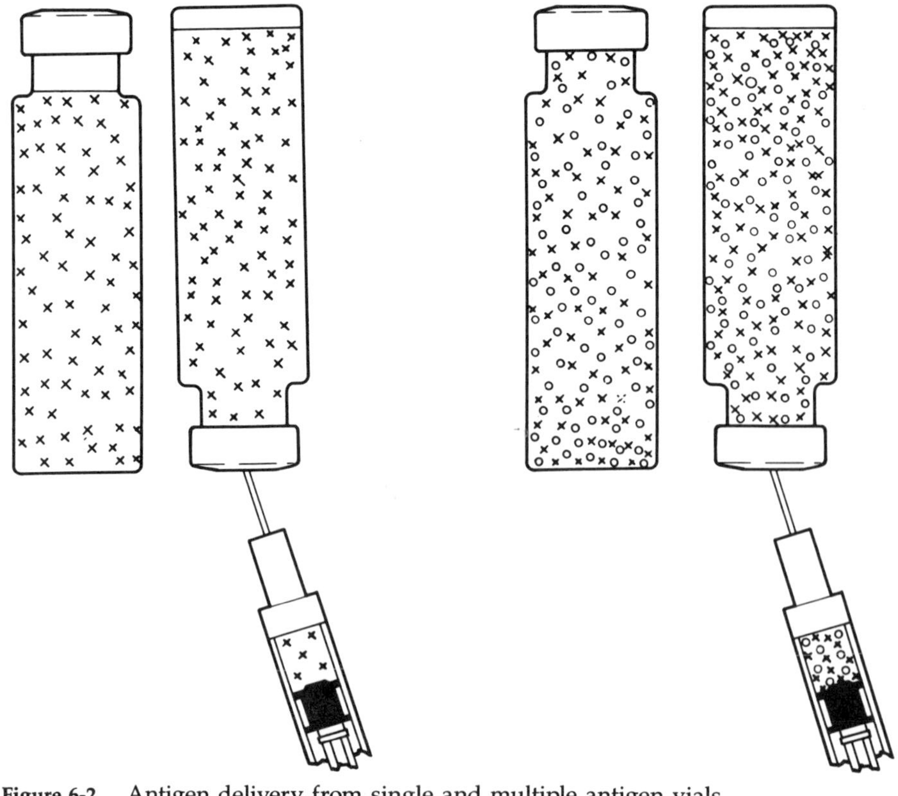

Figure 6-2. Antigen delivery from single and multiple antigen vials.

glycerine for stability. Additional glycerine is not added to vials on the testing board because it may produce confusing local reactions. However, a significant level of glycerine is needed in treatment vials to preserve their antigenicity. A 10% glycerine mixture used as a diluent is adequate to maintain antigenic potency for 3 months. (Since the antigens are in 50% glycerine, the actual glycerine level will actually be slightly greater than 10%.) If a commercially available 50% glycerine solution is diluted fivefold with diluent, the resulting 10% glycerine can be used as a diluent for the preparation of treatment vials. If glycerine is not added, vials will be potent for approximately 6 to 8 weeks, if refrigerated.

There is theoretically no limit to the number of antigens that may be combined in a single treatment vial. However, some practical considerations exist. For example, despite a bioassay (titration) to determine a safe starting point for therapy, antigens with very high endpoints must be advanced more cautiously than low endpoint antigens. Therefore, it is wise to employ initially at least two treatment vials, combining antigens of low endpoint (2 and 3) in one vial and antigens of high endpoint (4, 5, and 6) in another vial. If one or two antigens have especially high endpoints and the patient's history indicates marked sensitivity during these seasons, it is wise to treat such antigens separately. When maintenance doses are reached, as discussed in Chapter 7, all of the treatment antigens may usually be combined in a single vial without difficulty.

Suggested Readings

King HC. Endpoint titration and immunotherapy. *Otol Clin North Am* 1985;18(4):703–717.

King WP. The role of the skin end point titration method in allergy. In Goldman JL, ed. *The Principles and Practice of Rhinology*. New York: John Wiley & Sons, 1987:283–292.

· 7 ·

Immunotherapy Dosage Based on Skin Endpoint Titration

WALTER A. WARD, M.D., P.A., F.A.A.O.A.

After preparing the initial immunotherapy vial(s), it is best to administer the first dose in the office. If the patient is considered brittle or a hyperreactor, it would be prudent to vial test before the initial injection. (A brittle patient is an asthmatic or has experienced laryngospasm and/or angioedema.) Vial testing is done by intradermally injecting 0.01 cc from the immunotherapy vial to create a 4-mm wheal, and observing any resulting skin reaction after 10 minutes. A wheal size of 11 mm or less is considered acceptable, and the first treatment dose may then be injected. An intradermal test causing a wheal 13 mm in diameter should be considered the first treatment dose; the next dose, of 0.1 cc, is then given in 5 to 7 days, with subsequent escalation as noted below. If the wheal produced by the vial test is larger than 13 mm in diameter, "titrate the vial" by skin testing with progressively more dilute fivefold dilutions of the initial treatment vial until the resulting wheal is 11 mm or less. This antigen concentration is accepted as the initial treatment vial, and dose escalation proceeds.

There are two recommended methods for escalation of inhalant immunotherapy. For "brittle" or potentially hyperreactive patients, the initial dose is 0.05 cc, and this amount is increased by 0.05-cc increments every 5 to 7 days (e.g., 0.05, 0.1, 0.15, 0.2, etc.) until reaching a dose of 0.5 cc (Table 7-1). At this time, proceed to the next stronger treatment vial, containing each antigen one dilution more concentrated than the preceding one. For more stable or "nonbrittle" patients, immunotherapy can be advanced more rapidly, with an

Table 7-1. Initial Treatment Set

Schedule*			Schedule†	
Injection	*Amount (cc)*		*Injection*	*Amount (cc)*
1.	0.05		1.	0.05
2.	0.10		2.	0.10
3.	0.15		3.	0.20
4.	0.20	or	4.	0.30
5.	0.25		5.	0.40
6.	0.30		6.	0.50
7.	0.35			
8.	0.40			
9.	0.45			
10.	0.50			

*For therapist without long-term experience or for extremely sensitive patients.
†For experienced therapist or for less sensitive patients.

initial dose of 0.05 cc and a second one of 0.1 cc, but thereafter increased by increments of 0.1 cc every 5 to 7 days (e.g., 0.05, 0.1, 0.2, 0.3, etc.) until a dose of 0.5 cc is reached (Table 7-1). This schedule achieves hyposensitization much more rapidly.

The second treatment vial is normally prepared with each antigen five times more concentrated (one "dilution" stronger) than the initial treatment vial. This vial is antigenically five times more potent than the first treatment vial; thus, 0.1 cc is antigenically equivalent to 0.5 cc of the preceding vial. If 0.5 cc of the first vial was tolerated without reaction, 0.1 cc of the second vial should be a safe initial dose. Since the new vial is fresher, and theoretically slightly more potent antigenically, some individuals prefer to give a first dose of 0.05 cc from the new vial, and then proceed with dosage escalation as already described (Table 7-1).

Treatment vials are made progressively stronger, advancing toward the concentrate level, until a maintenance dose is reached. The maintenance dose is defined as one that causes a skin reaction less than the size of a half dollar (30 mm), while providing symptom relief for the greatest period of time (usually a week). It has been scientifically established that an antigen dose of 40 to 1000 μg (i.e., between 0.5 cc of the skin endpoint titration #4 dilution and 0.1 cc of the #1) is required for optimum production of blocking antibodies. However, control of the patient's symptoms is also important, and the dose that affords symptom relief for 7 days or more is also sought.

All allergists, no matter what their approach to immunotherapy, want to stop treatment just short of producing a systemic reaction. The use of skin endpoint titration (SET) minimizes this risk, by adjusting initial and subsequent antigen concentrations based on a bioassay in the individual patient. Further safety is assured by observing for skin reactions after each immunotherapy dose. Never advance an antigen dose if a local reaction 30 mm or larger (size of a half dollar) develops, and repeat the previous dose if the local reaction is 25 mm (size of a quarter).

Initially, it may be prudent to prepare two (or more) treatment vials, separating high reactors (endpoint #6, #5, #4) and low reactors (endpoint #3, #2). As various antigen strengths are advanced, vial contents may be combined as antigen levels approach one another, thereby eventually reducing the number of treatment vials to one (or two at most). Once the patient has reached a maintenance dose level and is asymptomatic, the period between injections may be lengthened. Most physicians give injections once or twice weekly until symptom relief lasts at least 7 days, and usually weekly injections are continued for at least 1 year. After that, depending on the patient, maintenance injection intervals may be lengthened to 2 and then 3 weeks. An interval between injections of greater than 3 weeks is not recommended, to reduce the risk of a reaction due to an amnestic response.

If, despite achieving treatment levels expected to achieve symptom relief, the patient remains symptomatic, it is imperative to consider the possible reasons. These might include:

1. Some antigens have been advanced to the concentrate or #1 dilution level, but other antigens in the treatment mix are not yet at sufficient strength to give symptom relief.
2. The dose given may be closer to a maximum tolerated dose than a symptom-relieving dose, representing overtreatment. Halve the current dose, then advance in 0.05-cc increments until the patient obtains relief of symptoms rather than an exacerbation of them.
3. The symptom-relieving dose was passed before the allergen came into season, and the current dose is too high. Either halve the current dose and advance in 0.05-cc increments until symptom relief is obtained (as above), or repeat SET for the suspected allergen to clarify the proper endpoint.
4. A concomitant food hypersensitivity is present. Suspect this if inhalant antigen therapy gives relief for only a few hours rather than days, or if symptoms flare postprandially or between 1:00 and 5:00 AM.
5. The immunotherapy mixture does not contain the allergen causing the symptoms. At this point, recheck the patient's history for clues to the offending antigen (minor pollens and molds, unusual epidermals, etc.), and for food and chemical hypersensitivities.
6. The antigen being given is not an active excitant of the patient's symptoms. Retitration or radioallergosorbent (RAST) testing may be helpful in clarifying this problem.

Conclusion

Allergists constantly strive for an immunotherapeutic dose that will relieve symptoms and build immunity while avoiding adverse reactions. At this time, I believe that the technique of SET is best suited for achieving this goal. The safety, even for high-dose immunotherapy, of treating with aliquots of the same material used for skin testing has been established by experience. Furthermore, SET enables testing and treatment to be carried out safely coseasonally, as well as beginning treatment preseasonally. Starting therapy at the endpoint of titration allows more rapid symptom control as well as significant economic savings to the patient and third-party payer.

Suggested Readings

King HC. Endpoint titration and immunotherapy. *Otolaryngol Clin North Am* 1985;18:703.

King WP. The role of the skin endpoint titration method in allergy. In Goldman J, ed. *The Principles and Practice of Rhinology*. New York: John Wiley & Sons, 1987.

Rinkel HJ. The management of clinical allergy, II: Etiologic factors and skin titration. *Arch Otolaryngol* 1963;77:56.

Ward WA. Skin endpoint titration immunotherapy. In Krause HF, ed. *Otolaryngic Allergy and Immunology*. Philadelphia: W.B. Saunders, 1989.

· 8 ·

Emergencies in the Allergy Office

JACK B. ANON, M.D., F.A.C.S., F.A.A.O.A.

Anaphylaxis in the allergy patient is probably one of the greatest fears for the neophyte as well as the seasoned allergist. This fear should always act as a constant reminder that problems can occur, but an understanding of what happens during anaphylaxis as well as an organized approach to the problem will allow the physician to deal safely with the emergency situation.

Anaphylaxis is a systemic hypersensitivity reaction that is immunologically mediated and induced by exposure to a specific antigen in a previously sensitized individual. The word anaphylaxis, which stems from the Greek term meaning "against protection," was originated by Porter and Richet in 1902 after they failed experimentally to produce prophylaxis to sea anemone toxin in dogs. These dogs were initially given low doses of the toxin in an attempt to vaccinate them against larger doses of the chemical. A repeat dose of the anemone extract injected several days later, however, led to rapid death, the exact opposite of the intended outcome.

There appear to be certain features that characterize the patients most likely to suffer an anaphylactic reaction. These include: a history of atopy, a family history of anaphylaxis, multiple exposures to the same or similar antigen, and the route of administration of the antigen (IV route vs. PO or IM).[1]

It is interesting to note that penicillin is the number one cause of death from anaphylaxis, with 300 cases reported per year, followed by *Hymenoptera* stings, which account for approximately 20 to 50 deaths per year.[2]

In this chapter we deal only with anaphylaxis after allergy testing or immunotherapy. The death toll from these were summarized in a 10-year retrospective study that showed that about 2.4 deaths per year are due to immunotherapy or skin testing. This is out of a projected 7 to 10 million allergen injections per year![3]

Pathophysiology

For the purpose of this discussion, we will refer only to Type I or immunoglobulin E (IgE)-mediated responses. Other types of anaphylaxis can occur, such as a reaction to iodinated x-ray contrast media, but this results from a direct action on the mast cell without an intermediate IgE step.[4] The non–immune-mediated reaction is termed *anaphylactoid*. The clinical picture of anaphylaxis versus anaphylactoid is indistinguishable.

In a Type I response, the body is exposed to the offending antigen, which links to the antigen-specific IgE attached to the mast cells. This leads to a change in the structure of the cell wall, thereby allowing calcium to enter the cell. During this phase of anaphylaxis, there is a release of preformed mediators via a degranulation process, as well as the synthesis of new compounds within the mast cell. The preformed mediators include histamine, proteases, heparin, proteoglycans, neutrophil chemotactic factor, eosinophil chemotactic factor, and acid hydrolases. The newly formed mediators are leukotrienes (also called slow-reacting substance of anaphylaxis),[5] bradykinin, serotonin, prostaglandins, and platelet-activating factor. These substances all have profound effects on the body that yield the many signs and symptoms of the anaphylactic reaction.

The major mediator, histamine, acts on the endothelial cells within arterioles, venules, and capillaries causing vessel dilation and increases in permeability. The subsequent loss of intravascular fluid through the permeable vessel, combined with peripheral pooling of fluid, leads to *hypovolemia and hypotension*, two major factors in anaphylactic shock. Leukotrienes (SRS-A) induce significant bronchospasm (up to 1000 times more potently than histamine), mucus production, and increased vascular permeability.[6] Eosinophil chemotactic factor is responsible for the many eosinophils seen in allergic reactions. Bradykinins are also potent bronchoconstricting agents.

Manifestations of Reaction

The body systems mainly involved in an anaphylactic reaction are the respiratory tract, cardiovascular, skin, gastrointestinal, genitourinary, and central nervous systems. The symptoms can range from a mild reaction to *rapid* death, with the usual finding that the sooner the symptoms begin after antigen exposure, the more severe the response.[7]

The mild reaction is heralded by a delayed onset, tingling sensation, flushing, tachycardia, sneezing, itching, some fullness of the throat, uneasiness, and diaphoresis. At this stage, the physician must differentiate between anaphylaxis and a vasovagal response. In contrast, the vasovagal response is characterized by bradycardia, pallor, no cutaneous symptoms, and nausea.

Moderate reactions are accompanied by the above findings plus bronchospasm, cough, shortness of breath, urticaria, and edema. Severe reactions include all of these features in a rapid fashion and to a more intense degree. Let us examine in detail the patient in moderate to severe anaphylaxis.

Within less than 30 minutes after receiving the offending allergen, skin reactions—the most common manifestation of anaphylaxis—will be observed.[8] The skin flushes and becomes warm to the touch as a result of histamine vasodilation. Small wheals along with larger areas of urticaria may be seen. Angioedema of the eyes, lips, tongue, and throat can also be found. Accompanying these signs is "angor animi": the sense by the patient of his impending doom (and at this point, the feeling is also shared by the physician!) (Fig. 8-1).

Another prominent finding is obstruction of the upper and lower airway. Edema in the upper respiratory tree will lead to dysphagia, stridor, and hoarseness in the laryngeal and supralaryngeal structures. Asthma due to bronchoconstriction along with increased mucus production will reduce the effectiveness of oxygenation and gas exchange in the bronchi. Approximately 70% of patients who die from anaphylaxis do so from respiratory complications.

Smooth muscle contractions are evidenced by nausea, stomach cramps, incontinence, and uterine cramping.

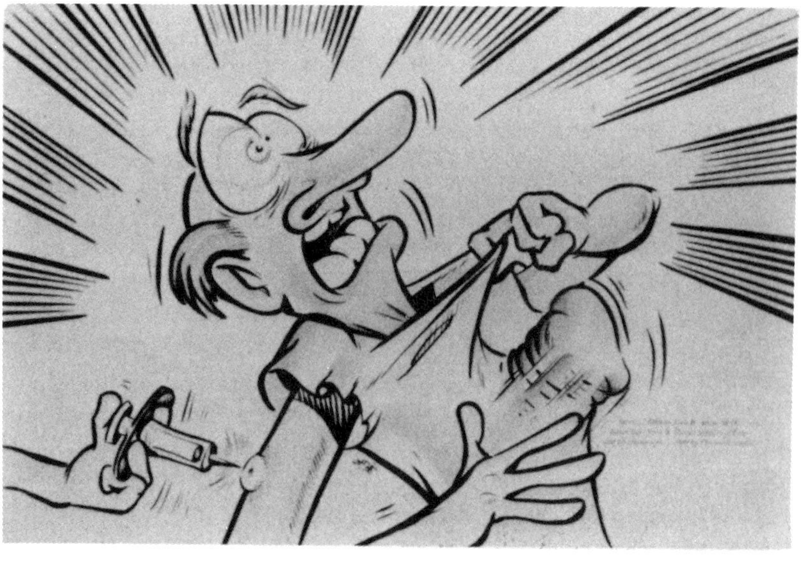

Figure 8-1. Illustration of severe anaphylactic reaction.

Cardiovascular collapse is a result of 1) hypovolemia from vasodilation, peripheral pooling, and extravasation of intravascular fluid, 2) depression of the myocardium by ischemia, and direct cardiotoxic effects of released mediators, 3) pulmonary vasoconstriction, and 4) arrhythmias secondary to sympathetic nervous stimulation. During the early compensatory stages of anaphylactic shock, the body attempts to override the decrease in blood pressure by increasing the heart rate and force of cardiac contraction (remember that stroke volume × heart rate = cardiac output). This accounts for the observed tachycardia. Systolic blood pressure can be maintained for a short while and, when accompanied by the rise in diastolic pressure, the pulse pressure will narrow.

Treatment

Immediate medical management is directed toward reducing the exposure to the antigen, reducing the effects of the chemical mediators, and instituting the ABC's of life support—airway, breathing, and circulation.

The steps to take during anaphylaxis are as follow. (Note that, while listed in a linear, numerical order, ideally more than one step should be performed simultaneously.)

1. **CALL FOR HELP!**
2. Intramuscular or subcutaneous injection of epinephrine 0.3 to 0.5 cc of a 1:1000 dilution.[9] This dose may be repeated every 10 to 15 minutes up to a maximum dose of 1.0 cc. The pediatric dose is 0.01 mg/kg of a 1:1000 dilution every 15 to 20 minutes. Prefilled spring loaded epinephrine "pens" are available and are prescribed for all patients who have had some type of anaphylactic reaction to stings (Fig. 8-2). Epinephrine has

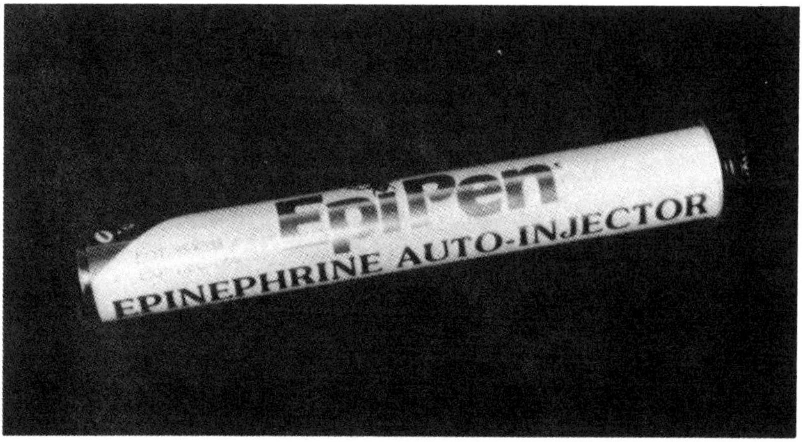

Figure 8-2. Prefilled epinephrine auto-injector syringe.

effects on both alpha and beta receptors. The alpha properties increase blood pressure, decrease peripheral vasodilation, and decrease the cutaneous manifestations of the reaction. The beta effects include bronchodilatation, positive inotropic and chronotropic changes on the heart, and increases in intracellular levels of cyclic adenosine monophosphate (AMP), which prevents further release of histamine and leukotrienes.[9]

Intravenous epinephrine in diluted form can be used in cases of severe cardiac collapse: 1 to 5 cc of 1:10,000 dilution for adults[10] and 0.01 to 0.05 cc/kg of 1:10,000 for children (Fig. 8-3). Be extremely cautious, for this route of administration can be very dangerous!

Last, if an intravenous (IV) route cannot be started, injection into the tongue or into an endotracheal tube gives IV drug levels.[2]

3. Apply a tourniquet above the injection site to slow absorption of the injected antigen. Remember to loosen every 15 minutes!
4. Place a blood pressure cuff on the arm opposite the injection site and monitor the pressure frequently.

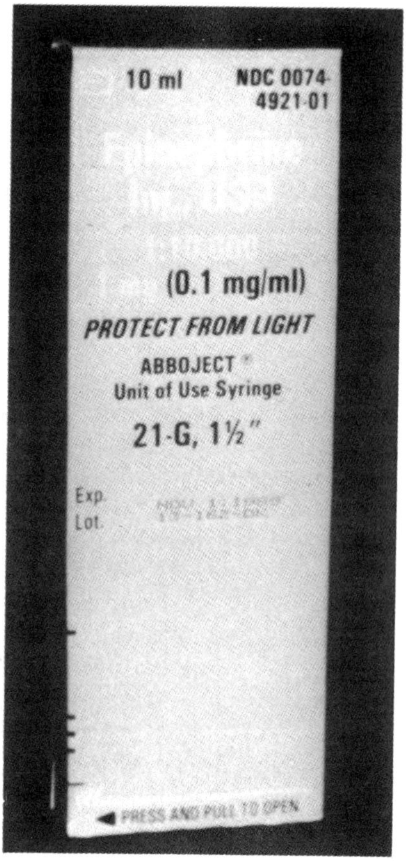

Figure 8-3. Intravenous 1:10,000 epinephrine.

5. If in shock, place the head down and the feet up to improve blood return. This position is not recommended if the airway is compromised.
6. Establish an IV line quickly with a large-bore needle (ideally provided by a 14-gauge catheter in the antecubital region). Vascular collapse can make it difficult to find veins if this step is delayed! Fluid replacement should begin as rapidly as possible. Squeezing the IV bag can give a fast fluid flow. The IV fluid should be normal saline or Ringer's solution. If a hypotonic fluid is given it tends to exit the vessels too rapidly. Use blood pressure as a guide to fluid volume. *N.B.*: be careful not to fluid overload the elderly patient, or a patient with a history of congestive heart failure.
7. Oxygen should be started by mask or Ambu-bag® (Fig. 8-4). If upper airway obstruction becomes a problem, then intubation or cricothyrotomy may be necessary (Fig. 8-5). Lower airway obstruction can be relieved by the administration of orally inhaled albuterol or other beta agonist oral inhalers. Airway management will also be aided by the availability of an efficient suction apparatus to deal with the thick mucus provided in the respiratory tree. It is useless to establish an airway only to find it plugged with mucus!
8. Antihistamines play a strong role in the competitive binding of those sites that have yet to bind histamine. There is no effect on already bound sites.

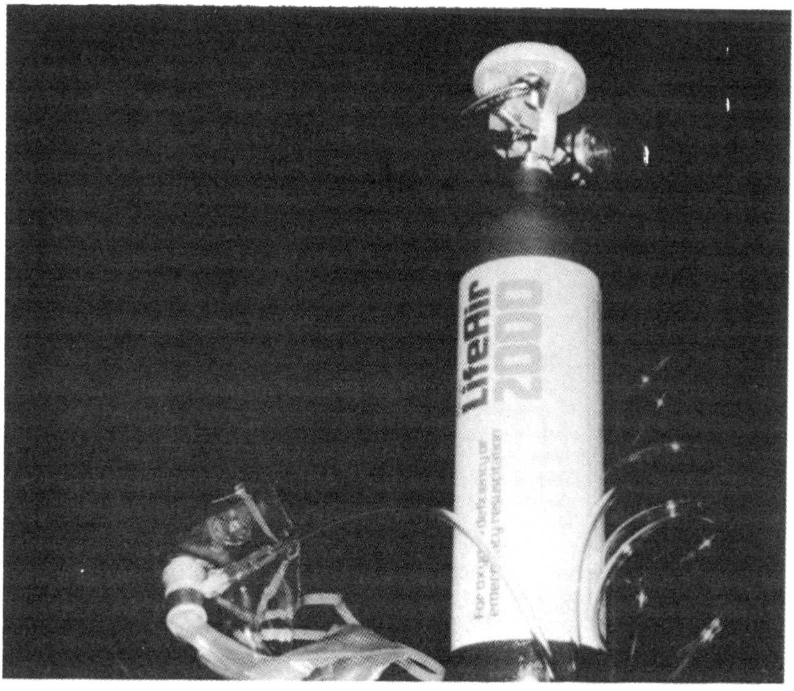

Figure 8-4. Oxygen tank with attached face mask.

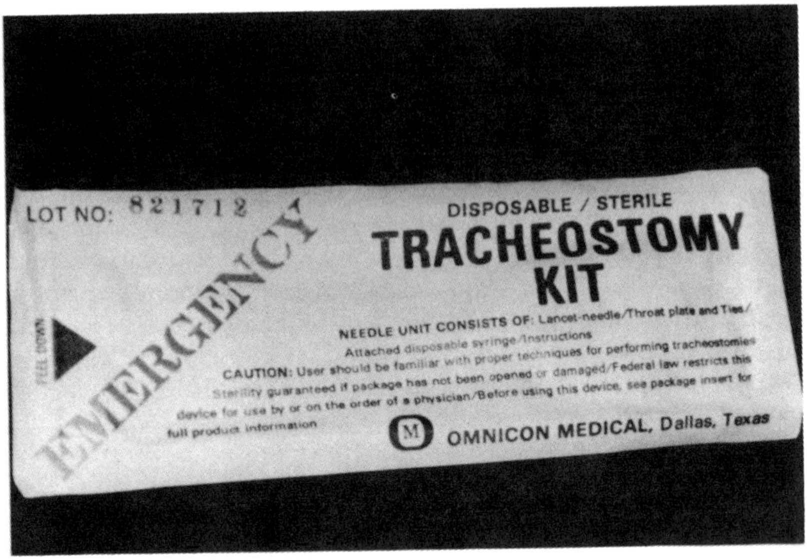

Figure 8-5. Emergency cricothyrotomy/tracheostomy device.

The drug most commonly administered is diphenhydramine. The usual dose is 50 to 100 mg IV or intramuscularly (IM). The pediatric dose is 5 mg/kg/24 h in divided doses.

9. Steroids play no role in the immediate anaphylactic period, but are important in preventing delayed reactions. Hydrocortisone 250 to 500 mg intravenous push (IVP) (4–8 mg/kg children) or dexamethasone 8 mg IVP should be given.
10. IV or IM H_2 inhibitors such as ranitidine can be beneficial in blocking hypotension and improving cardiac function. Dosage is 50 mg IM or 50 mg diluted in 20 cc of saline given in a period greater than 2 minutes IV.[8]
11. If hypotension is refractory to epinephrine, then other vasopressor agents such as dopamine are required. This can be diluted by adding 5 cc of the 80 mg/cc vial to 500 cc of IV solution. Dopamine must have a separate IV line because it precipitates with many medications, especially aminophylline. The rate of administration is determined by the response of the blood pressure. Dopamine is effective only when hypovolemia is also corrected with IV fluids.
12. Aminophylline inhibits the degradation of cyclic AMP, thus decreasing the release of mediators.[11] There may also be a direct positive action on the heart muscle. The bronchodilator effects are well known, but because aminophylline may worsen hypotension, this drug should be used only to relieve bronchospasm when epinephrine has failed to work. The dose is 6 mg/kg IV over 30 minutes followed by a 0.5 to 0.8 mg/kg/h drip.[12]
13. Besides the above drugs, heparin 10,000 USP units should be given early in the course of the reaction. Dolowitz has shown that the acid polysac-

charide heparin can neutralize histamine by detoxification as well as by direct binding to the alkaline histamine, which produces a neutral salt.[13]

It is important to identify all patients in an allergy practice who are on beta blockers before testing is undertaken. Patients who are undergoing immunotherapy and are started on beta blockers need to notify the allergy office. This is an important point, because anaphylactic shock in these patients is anecdotally reported to be severe and refractory to treatment by epinephrine. This is because epinephrine produces alpha, beta 1, and beta 2 agonist effects. If there is a beta blocker on board, especially a noncardioselective drug such as propranolol, then there will be a preference of the epinephrine to affect the alpha pathway. This can be quite detrimental, as the enhanced alpha activity can dramatically increase the blood pressure response to epinephrine, with a resultant hypertensive crisis.

If anaphylaxis occurs in a patient on a beta blocker, epinephrine can be used as described above if the blood pressure is closely monitored. Heparin can also be administered. The application of MAST trousers (obviously by the paramedic) has been shown to be effective in treating shock.[14] The use of glucagon has also been reported: its mechanism of action is felt to be an increase in cyclic AMP within the cell, thus blocking the release of mediators.[11]

Epinephrine should also be administered cautiously to patients taking tricyclic antidepressants and monoamine oxidase inhibitors, as these drugs will potentiate its effect, resulting in tachycardia and hypertension.

In the unlikely event a hypertensive crisis ensues with the above, then an infusion of IV nitroprusside can be started, 0.25 μg/kg/min to 8 μg/kg/min titrated according to the blood pressure.[15]

As can be seen, the treatment of anaphylaxis requires a step-by-step approach to the problem. This chapter serves only as a guide to the use of the various drugs and techniques. It is recommended that each allergist review these emergency procedures with the members of the allergy staff. Take time to run a drill with the staff to identify areas of possible problems, such as, where will the patient be placed for all of the above treatment? Where will the IV bag be hung? Are there enough needles and syringes? How does the oxygen tank connect? Is the oxygen tank always full? Where is the suction machine plugged in? Do the suction catheters fit through the cricothyrotomy unit? Do not rely solely on prepacked kits such as the Banyan. They are often missing key drugs, have drugs that are not needed, or the instruments may not be adequate.

Emergency Procedures

1. **CALL FOR HELP!**
2. Patient recumbent, elevate legs, loosen clothing.
3. Ammonia for vasovagal response. Oxygen as needed.
4. Apply tourniquet above site, loosen q15 min, BP cuff on opposite arm.

Check vital signs. Vagal—slow pulse, clammy; anaphylactic—rapid pulse, flushing.

5. Epinephrine 0.3–0.5 cc IM or SQ every 10–15 minutes.
6. Airway management as needed. Albuterol inhalers, one puff every minute up to 6 puffs maximum. Stop if significant tachycardia or tremor occurs. Intubation or tracheotomy with adequate suction available.
7. Begin IV with large-bore needle. Rapid fluid infusion: squeeze bag for faster flow rate. Be careful in patients with a history of CHF.
8. Diphenhydramine 50–100 mg IVP.
9. Hydrocortisone 250 mg IVP.
10. Ranitidine 50 mg IM or 50 mg diluted with normal saline to 20 cc IV given over 5-minute infusion.
11. Dopamine 5 cc of 80 mg/cc vial to 500 cc fluid. Give as needed to titrate BP (need separate IV line from Aminophylline).
12. Heparin 10,000 USP units IVP.
13. Aminophylline 6 mg/kg IV over 30 minutes followed by 0.2–1.0 mg/kg/h drip (recommended for hospital setting only).

Acknowledgments

I would like to thank B. Barnes, M.D., and David Race, M.D., Department of Emergency Medicine, Saint Vincent Health Center, as well as B. Staszak, R.N., for reviewing this chapter.

References

1. Stoelting RK. Allergic reactions during anesthesia. *Anesth Analg* 1983;62:341–356.
2. Lucke WC, Thomas, H. Anaphylaxis: Pathophysiology, clinical presentations and treatment. *J Emerg Med* 1983;1:83–95.
3. Lockey RF, Benedict LM, Turkeltaub PC, Bukantz SC. Fatalities from immunotherapy (IT) and skin testing (ST). *J Allergy Clin Immunol* 1987;79(4):660–677.
4. Sheffer AL, Pennoyer DS. Management of adverse drug reactions. *J Allergy Clin Immunol* 1984;74(4):580–588.
5. Lockey RF, Bukantz SC. *Fundamentals of Immunology and Allergy*. Philadelphia: W.B. Saunders, 1987.
6. Mygind N. *Essential Allergy: An Illustrated Text for Students and Specialists*. Blackwell Publishing, 1986.
7. Netzel MC. Anaphylaxis: clinical presentation, immunologic mechanisms, and treatment. *J Emerg Med* 1986;4:227–236.
8. Bierman CW, Pearlman DS. *Allergic Diseases from Infancy to Adulthood*, 2nd ed. Philadelphia: W.B. Saunders, 1988:672–674.
9. Barach EM, Nowad RM, Lee TG, Tomlanovich MC. Epinephrine for treatment of anaphylactic shock. *JAMA* 1984;251(16):2118–2122.
10. Terr AI. Anaphylaxis. *Clin Rev Allergy* 1985;3:3–23.
11. Perkin RM, Anas NG. Mechanisms and management of anaphylactic shock not responding to traditional therapy. *Ann Allergy* 1985;54:202–208.
12. Guill, MF. Allergy emergencies. *Immunol Allergy Clin North Am* 1987;7(3):485–500.
13. Dolowitz DA, Dougherty TF. The use of heparin in the control of allergies. *Ann Allergy* 1965;23:309–313.
14. Bickell WH, Dice WH. Military antishock trousers in a patient with adrenergic-resistant anaphylaxis. *Ann Emerg Med* 1984;13(3):189–190.
15. Drugs for hypertensive emergencies. *Med Lett Drugs Therapeut* 1989;31:32–34.

Appendix 1

Glossary

The material presented here should help the novice to comprehend many of the terms used in skin endpoint titration and otolaryngic allergy in general. Because of space limitations, the definitions are at times simplistic. For more details, the reader is referred to the chapters in this text, to the other excellent texts on otolaryngic allergy that are available, and to the sponsored and approved courses of the AAOA.

Richard L. Mabry, M.D., F.A.C.S., F.A.A.O.A.

Acute Phase Reaction: In a Gell and Coombs type I (anaphylactic) reaction, the initial allergic response, mediated by preformed and newly formed mediators of inflammation released from mast cells and basophils.

Allergy: The production of symptoms through immunologic mechanisms by a substance that is not harmful in itself.

Anaphylaxis: An immunologically mediated, immediate-type, multisystem reaction that is often severe and sometimes lethal.

Antibody: Specific immunoglobulin produced in response to a stimulus by an antigen.

Antigen: A substance capable of eliciting a response by the immune system, producing a substance (antibody) specific to the challenging substance.

Antigen Screen: A limited number of allergens used in initial testing (*in vivo* or *in vitro*) in order to identify allergic individuals most efficiently.

Antihistamine: A drug that controls allergic symptoms (e.g., rhinorrhea, itching) by competing with histamine for H1 receptor sites.

Basophil: A leukocyte, the granules of which stain blue, that participates in some types of acute allergic reactions.

Beta-Blocker: A drug most often used in the management of hypertension and vascular headaches that blocks beta-adrenergic stimuli and may complicate allergy skin testing and immunotherapy.

Bevel: The slanted portion of a hypodermic needle.

Concentrate: Antigen, as obtained from the supplier, in extremely concentrated form, and usually containing 50% glycerine as a preservative. (Also called "Stock Vial.")

Corticosteroid: A drug (glucocorticoid) with potent antiinflammatory effects that alleviates the symptoms of an allergic reaction while providing protection from the late phase reaction.

Cromolyn: A drug that stabilizes mast cells, preventing both acute and late phase allergic reactions by inhibiting mast cell degranulation and the resulting release of mediators of inflammation.

Cross-Reactivity: The ability of more than one antigen to react with a specific antibody, due to similar or identical antigen–antibody combining sites (called epitopes).

Decongestant: An alpha-adrenergic drug used (topically or systemically) in pharmacotherapy to produce shrinkage of congested nasal mucosa.

Diluent: The (usually) antigenically inert substance (e.g., phenolated saline) used for volume adjustment in the preparation of various concentrations of antigenic materials.

Endpoint: In skin endpoint titration, the antigenic concentration at which progressive positive whealing first occurs.

Eosinophil: A leukocyte, the granules of which stain red, that participates in the allergic reaction (most often in the late phase), and is found in increased numbers in the peripheral blood and nasal secretions of allergic individuals.

Epidermal Antigen: An allergen associated with the skin (fur, etc.) of animals (e.g., cat dander).

Flash Response: A variant response in skin endpoint titration in which a series of negative responses is suddenly followed by a large positive wheal.

Fungi: A large class of vegetable organisms (e.g., mushrooms, toadstools), which includes molds.

Gell and Coombs Reactions: Classifications of allergic reactions according to the mechanisms involved (e.g., Gell and Coombs type I reaction, which is IgE-mediated, immediate, and exemplified by anaphylaxis).

Glycerine: A preservative contained in most antigen stock vials (usually in a 50% concentration) to extend the useful life of the biologic material.

Glycerine Control: Application of a 4-mm wheal of 2% glycerine, for comparison with skin reactions obtained with a #2 antigen concentration (which normally also contains 2% glycerine).

Histamine: A mediator of inflammation that plays an important role in the acute allergic response.

Histamine Control: Creation of a 4-mm wheal using dilute histamine to demonstrate a positive reaction and confirm the presence of an intact wheal-and-flare response.

Immunoglobulin: Human serum globulin produced as a consequence of antigenic stimulation; classified as immunoglobulins (Ig) M, A, D, G, and E.

Immunotherapy: Regular injections with appropriate allergens to produce tolerance in the host through varied immunologic mechanisms, including an eventual drop in allergen-specific IgE and a rise in IgG ("blocking antibodies").

Inhalant Allergy: Allergy to a substance that enters the body via the respiratory tract (as opposed to hypersensitivity to ingested material or "food allergy").

Intracutaneous Testing: Another term for intradermal testing.

Intradermal Testing: Injection of a test antigen just under the outermost layer of epidermis to form a wheal.

***In Vitro* Testing**: (literally, testing "in glass") Testing (for allergy) by laboratory means, such as RAST or ELISA testing.

***In Vivo* Testing**: (literally, testing "in life") Testing (for allergy) by skin testing methods, such as prick-puncture, intradermal, or skin endpoint titration testing.

Late Phase Reaction: In a Gell and Coombs type I (anaphylactic) reaction, the phase that follows the acute phase by 4 to 6 hours.

Linear Testing: Skin endpoint titration in which testing for a single antigen is accomplished by placing wheals using progressively more concentrated antigen strengths until the endpoint is determined by the formation of a positive wheal followed by a confirming wheal.

Mast Cell: A cell found in respiratory and connective tissue that releases preformed and newly formed mediators of inflammation (e.g., histamine) as part of acute (anaphylactic) allergic reactions.

Molds: A type of fungi, also called *fungi imperfecta*, having septate mycelia; numerous molds are potential allergens (e.g., Aspergillus, Cladosporium).

Multiple Dose Vial: A treatment vial containing sufficient quantity for the withdrawal and administration of several immunotherapy injections.

Multitest: A puncture test using a multipronged device for introducing multiple antigens (plus a positive and negative control) with a single application.

Negative Control: A skin test wheal made using only diluent without added antigen, to rule out primary skin hyperreactivity.

Perennial Allergens: Allergens that are present virtually year-round (e.g., animal danders, molds).

Plateau Reaction: A skin whealing response during skin endpoint titration in which two (or more) of the positive wheals are the same size.

Pollen: A potential allergen source, composed of fertilizing elements of a flowering plant.

Prick Test: A skin test in which the skin is punctured at a 45° angle, through a drop of antigen, introducing a small amount into the skin.

Prick-Puncture Test: A variant of the prick test in which the puncture through the antigen droplet is vertical to the skin surface.

Seasonal Allergens: Allergens that are present during specific periods of the year (e.g., ragweed in the fall).

SET: (Skin endpoint titration, formerly called serial dilution endpoint titration) Intradermal skin testing that is begun with an anticipated nonreacting antigen dilution, continuing with fivefold stronger concentrations to determine the concentration at which progressive positive skin responses occur (i.e., the "endpoint of titration").

Single Dose Vial: A treatment vial containing the exact amount for one immunotherapy injection.

Standardized Extract: Antigen the biologic potency of which is expressed in comparison with standards developed by an overseeing body (e.g., World Health Organization).

Stock Vial: Antigen, as obtained from the supplier, in extremely concentrated form, and usually containing 50% glycerine as a preservative (also called "Concentrate").

Testing Board: A collection of relevant antigens in varying concentrations [usually 1:100 (#1) to 1:312,500 (#6)] and with no added glycerine, used for skin testing.

Titration: A bioassay involving the application of progressively stronger antigen concentrations to determine the point at which reactivity is first noted.

"Titrate The Vial": Diluting the contents of an antigen-containing treatment vial by fivefold increments, then making test wheals with these concentrations to determine a safe starting point for dosage (used mainly when vials formulated from *in vitro* testing yield an unacceptably large vial test wheal).

TOE: Term for three species of fungi [*Trichophyton, Epidermophyton* and *Oidomycetes* (*Candida*)] that are responsible for a delayed hypersensitivity reaction with frequent cutaneous manifestations.

Treatment Board: A collection of relevant antigens in varying concentrations [usually 1:20 (concentrate) to 1:12,500 (#4)], often mixed using 10% glycerine for stability, used to prepare treatment vials.

Treatment Vial: A mixture of relevant allergens (to which the patient has been demonstrated to be allergic) in appropriate concentrations for administration of immunotherapy.

Vertical Testing: A screening maneuver in which skin testing for several antigens is done simultaneously, starting with the #6 concentration, then (if necessary) the #4 and #2 dilutions to estimate the degree of sensitivity present. (The definitive endpoint may accurately be determined by linear testing.)

Vial Test: Making a skin wheal with material from a treatment vial to determine if the concentrations of antigen are appropriate (and safe) for commencing immunotherapy. This type of test must *always* precede initial immunotherapy based on *in vitro* results.

W/V Concentration: Antigen strength expressed as grams of antigen per milliliter of extracting fluid.

Wheal: In allergy, an elevated area on the skin surface, initially produced by an intradermal injection, the ultimate size of which is also affected by cutaneous hypersensitivity and other factors.

Appendix 2

Patient Information

The following material is furnished through the courtesy of Dr. Helen F. Krause, to supplement the information contained in her chapter in this monograph (Chapter 1). The AAOA appreciates the efforts of Dr. Krause in providing this information. Each individual clinician will wish to adapt the material presented here to fit the individual circumstances of his/her practice and should bear in mind that nothing in medicine can be done according to a uniform "cookbook" routine that will fit every situation.

Richard L. Mabry, M.D., F.A.C.S., F.A.A.O.A.

For Our Patients

As a patient in our office, you have consulted us for evaluation of your ear, nose, or throat problem. There is an indication that your health problem is caused by or seriously affected by allergic disease. You may be considering an allergic evaluation (tests, etc.) in our office. We have prepared the following information for you so that you may be better informed before you decide to undertake the expense and time required for proper allergic evaluation.

What Are Allergies?

Common allergic problems that are easily recognized are "hay fever" and asthma. Skin eruptions from food ingestion (e.g., hives from strawberries and eczema from chocolate) are also commonly recognized as allergic problems. More recently, medical investigators have demonstrated that many common and puzzling ear, nose, and throat problems may be the result of chronic allergy.

Allergies are sensitivities that susceptible persons develop to normally harmless substances. The tendency to become susceptible to various things in our environment is usually inherited. Parents frequently deny any knowledge of allergy in the family history, but further questioning will usually reveal patterns of food intolerances, "sinus trouble," and other changes to suggest long-standing, although mild, allergic disease. If the susceptibility to allergy is inherited, then it is the amount of exposure to an offending substance (allergen) that will determine whether the individual will develop a severe illness as a result of his allergy, or will only be aware of mild changes. The greater the time and/or amount of exposure, the greater the chances that a susceptible person will develop an allergic problem that will require medical management.

Allergens are substances that are capable of producing allergy. When an allergen enters the body, substances called antibodies are produced. The interaction of the allergen and the antibody produce an irritation in the affected tissue. The swelling of the nasal lining during the hay fever season would be an example of this interaction.

Allergens may enter the body by ingestion, inhalation, injection, and by external contact with the skin. It is then apparent that foods, dust, pollens, fumes, and almost anything in the environment may cause allergic diseases. In testing for allergy, emphasis is placed on the two most important groups: foods and inhalants (dust, pollens, and molds). Methods for detecting allergy to other substances are also available.

Allergy Tests

There are several ways to test for allergies: the scratch test, punch or prick test, inhalation and ingestion tests, intradermal tests and RAST (radioallergosorbent test) done on the patient's blood sample. In our office, we do titration testing using the intradermal method and the RAST method, because we feel they are the most scientific and the safest procedures available. We have multiple dilutions of our allergens that are used in testing. The intradermal test is made by injecting a minute amount of allergen just under the skin. The resulting wheal resembles a small mosquito bite and after 10 minutes of observation, an increase in size generally indicates a positive reaction to that dilution. The number of tests required will depend on a patient's detailed history and on the test reactions. RAST involves taking a sample of blood from the patient and using a sophisticated laboratory procedure for allergy determination. A few intradermal skin tests are then used to correlate the results and institute treatment. Several techniques are available to test for food allergies also. All treatments will be explained in detail if you are to undergo allergy testing.

By establishing the endpoint dilution, we are able to reach the level of optimum relief of allergic symptoms more rapidly. We are also able to recheck the endpoint dilution when we fail to obtain optimum relief in a reasonable period.

Treatment

Treatment of allergy is a cooperative venture with both patient and physician as participants. The goal of treatment is to produce an allergic balance so that the patient may be freed of existing allergic illness and avoid the development of new allergic problems. A basic part of management is teaching the patient to eliminate offending allergens whenever possible. Since certain allergens cannot be eliminated, the reaction of the patient to these substances is controlled by desensitization.

Desensitization is the technique of injecting small but increasing amounts of the allergen to control the allergic reaction so that the patient has little or no reaction when he is exposed to the offending substance. In our office, desensitization by injection is used for inhalant allergens. Food sensitivities can be dealt with by diet control or skin testing. In conjunction with desensitization, patients will be taught to avoid and eliminate allergens.

Allergy History Questionnaire

NAME ____________ REFERRED BY ________ DATE ________
ADDRESS ____________
TELEPHONE: HOME ______ WORK ______ EMPLOYER ________
BIRTHDATE ______ AGE ______ MARITAL STATUS ______
INSURANCE INFORMATION: NAME OF INSURED ________
EMPLOYER OF INSURED ____________
INSURANCE COMPANY ________ INSURANCE NUMBERS ______

PLEASE STUDY CAREFULLY EACH QUESTION AND ANSWER IT AS BEST YOU CAN:

YES NO

____ ____ COUGH? Constant ____ Intermittent ____ Daytime ____ Nighttime ____
____ ____ FREQUENT COLDS OR UPPER RESPIRATORY INFECTIONS ____ AS A CHILD ____
____ ____ TEMPERATURE WITH COLDS?
____ ____ SNEEZING?
What might precipitate it or increase it? ________
Is it seasonal or related to location? ________
____ SORE THROATS? Frequency? ________
From infections? YES ____ NO ____
From drainage? YES ____ NO ____
____ ____ NOSE DRAINAGE? From the front or down the throat? Circle one.
Drainage clear or colored? Thick? ____ Thin? ____ From right side ____ Left ____
____ ____ NOSE BLOCKAGE? Right side ____ Left side ____
Both sides? ____
____ ____ EYE SYMPTOMS? Burning, puffy, watering? Circle one.
Itching? YES ____ NO ____ Where? Inside corner ____ Outside corner ____ All over ____
____ ____ HEADACHES? Which part of head? ________
What starts a headache? ________
What makes it worse? ________
Is headache worse at any time of day? ________
Can you tell when a headache may be starting? ____ How? ______
____ ____ FATIGUE? When? Certain times of the day? ____ Before eating? ____ After eating? ____ Certain days of the week? ____ When?
____
Chronic (all of the time) ________
____ ____ Shortness of breath/Do you know why? Explain ________
____ ____ WHEEZING? Now? ____ As a child? ____ With exercise? ____
Out in the cold? ____ With infections? ____
Other things that cause your wheezing? ________
____ ____ ASTHMA? Now? ____ As a child? ____
____ ____ AS A CHILD DID YOU HAVE FREQUENT URINARY TRACT INFECTIONS?

YES	NO	
_____	_____	DO YOU HAVE "SINUS PROBLEMS"?
_____	_____	EARACHES? Do your ears drain or run? _____ If so, clear or cloudy drainage? Do you experience any of the following sounds or sensations? Itchy? _____ Stuffy? _____ Flaky? _____ Ring? _____ Buzz? _____ Crackle? _____ Pop? _____ Other sounds? _____ Hearing loss? _____
_____	_____	VERTIGO (DIZZINESS)? When? __________
_____	_____	LOSS OF SMELL? When? __________
_____	_____	LOSS OF TASTE? When? __________
_____	_____	LARYNGITIS?
_____	_____	ECZEMA? Now? _____ As a child? _____ Describe type and location __________
_____	_____	HIVES? When? _____ Where? _____ Specify: _____ Any known material that causes a rash? __________ Soap? _____ Ointments? _____ Paint? _____ Clothing? _____ Cosmetics? _____ Poison Ivy? _____
_____	_____	FUNGUS INFECTIONS? Athletes foot? _____ Vaginitis? _____ Jock Rash? _____
_____	_____	DO YOU CURRENTLY HAVE PREMENSTRUAL SYNDROME (Female)?
_____	_____	DO YOU HAVE ACNE?
_____	_____	HAVE YOU EVER BEEN DIAGNOSED AS HAVING ENDOMETRIOSIS? (Female)
_____	_____	PETS? Kind? _____ Kept inside or outside? _____ Breed? _____ How long have you had your pet? _____ Symptoms worse when visiting friends who have pets? YES _____ NO _____ Animal contact that causes symptoms? _____
_____	_____	DO YOU SMOKE? Cigarettes? _____ Cigars? _____ Pipe? _____ Chew tobacco? _____ Snuff? _____
_____	_____	IF YOU DO NOT SMOKE, DOES SOMEONE ELSE'S SMOKE BOTHER YOU?
_____	_____	DO YOU PERSPIRE EXCESSIVELY?
_____	_____	DO YOU REGARD YOURSELF AS BEING NERVOUS?
_____	_____	Problem with personality or behavioral changes? Certain times of the day? Explain: _____ Certain seasons? _____ With certain foods? __________
_____	_____	ITCHINESS? Nose? _____ Roof of mouth? _____ Ears? _____ Hands? _____ Feet? _____
_____	_____	WERE YOU A PREMATURE BABY?
_____	_____	As an infant, were you taken off formula or any foods? Specify: __________
_____	_____	Were you a colicky or fussy baby? Breast- or bottle-fed? Circle one.
_____	_____	HAVE YOU EVER EXPERIENCED ANXIETY OR PANIC ATTACKS?
_____	_____	Are you being treated?
_____	_____	Do you suspect any food of increasing your symptoms? Specify: __________
_____	_____	Do you have any specific cravings or do you overindulge in certain foods? List: __________

YES NO

_____ _____ Does any certain food give you indigestion, hives, or otherwise upset you? Specify: ______________________________

_____ _____ DO YOU HAVE IRRITABLE BOWEL?

_____ _____ Do you have excess gas without eating gaseous foods, such as fiber, beans, cabbage, etc.?

_____ _____ Are you awakened during the night with any symptoms? Which symptoms?
Headaches? _____ Bloating? _____ Dizziness? _____ Thirst? _____
Stomach cramps? _____ Heartburn? _____ Dry cough? _____
Sore throat? _____

_____ _____ Do you awaken in the morning with any symptoms?
Joint pain/stiffness _____ Increased congestion? _____
Increased drainage _____ Nausea _____ Other? _____

DO YOUR SYMPTOMS INCREASE OR DECREASE WITH THE FOLLOWING CONDITIONS:

INCREASE	DECREASE	SAME	
_____	_____	_____	Cold weather
_____	_____	_____	Warm weather
_____	_____	_____	Air conditioning
_____	_____	_____	Windy days
_____	_____	_____	March to May
_____	_____	_____	May to July
_____	_____	_____	August to October
_____	_____	_____	November to March
_____	_____	_____	Damp weather
_____	_____	_____	Housework (dusting, etc.)
_____	_____	_____	High pollution levels
_____	_____	_____	Change of seasons
_____	_____	_____	When furnace goes on
_____	_____	_____	Going to bed
_____	_____	_____	After asleep for a short time
_____	_____	_____	Upon arising
_____	_____	_____	Later in day, 4 to 9 PM
_____	_____	_____	Being in or mowing grass

HOME AND WORK ENVIRONMENT
(Please Specify by H for Home and W for Work)
What is your occupation? ______________________________
Do you participate in any particular activities, hobbies, or recreation? __________
Please Specify: ______________________________
Are your symptoms increased at home, work or no change? (circle one)
Are you exposed to excessive amounts of dusts, fumes, chemicals, noise? __________
Are there plants, dried flowers, fresh flowers at home or work? __________
HEATING SYSTEM: (HOME AND WORK)
Electric _____ Gas _____ Oil _____ Propane _____ Kerosene heater _____ Forced air _____ Hot water _____ Fireplace _____ Wood burning stove _____ Coal burning stove _____ Air conditioning _____ Air cleaner _____ Humidifier _____
COOKING: Gas _____ Electric _____ Propane _____

LAUNDRY: Do you use softener sheets, liquid softener, or bleach in laundry? Circle one.

COSMETICS:

Do you use make-up? _____ eye make-up _____ perfume _____ aftershave _____

HOUSING:

Do you live in a house? _____ Two story _____ Split level _____ Ranch _____ Trailer _____

Do you live in an apartment? _____ Small building _____ Large building _____ Older building _____ Newer building _____

Have you had insulation blown into your house? ______________________________

FURNITURE:

Upholstered _____ Not upholstered _____

Fabric _____ Vinyl _____ Other (What) ______________________________

FLOOR COVERINGS:

_____ Carpeting and pads
_____ Carpets and pads
_____ Rugs and pads
_____ Throw rugs
_____ Linoleum

WALL COVERINGS:

_____ Wallpaper
_____ Fabric
_____ Paneling
_____ Tapestries
_____ Pennants

MATTRESS:

_____ Innerspring
_____ Waterbed
_____ Foam rubber
_____ Other (Specify)

____

WINDOW COVERINGS

_____ Washable curtains/drapes
_____ Unwashable curtains/drapes
_____ Shades
_____ Blinds
_____ Others

BEDS AND BEDDING

_____ Number of beds (your room)
_____ Comforters
_____ Chenille bedspread
_____ Stuffed animals

PILLOWS:

_____ Feather or down
_____ Foam rubber
_____ Kapok
_____ Dacron or polyester

Do your symptoms improve, get worse or stay the same when on vacation? Circle one.

Where do you usually go on vacation? Mountains, Seashore, Other ______________

FAMILY HISTORY:

Have any of your blood relatives had any of the following illnesses? If so, underline and check the relationship.

	FATHER	MOTHER	BROTHER	SISTER	CHILD
BRONCHIAL ASTHMA	________	________	________	________	________
EMPHYSEMA	________	________	________	________	________
HAY FEVER	________	________	________	________	________
SINUS PROBLEMS	________	________	________	________	________
HIVES	________	________	________	________	________
POSTNASAL DRAINAGE	________	________	________	________	________
ECZEMA	________	________	________	________	________
THYROID PROBLEMS	________	________	________	________	________
FOOD ALLERGIES	________	________	________	________	________

How long have you had specific symptoms that brought you to our office? _____ Years _____ Months _____ Weeks _____ Days

Have you had allergy testing before?
Doctor who performed the tests ________________ Address ______________
Date last testing ________ Type of testing: Scratch, Intradermal, RAST (Circle one)
Were there positive reactions? _____ To what? ______________________
Were you treated? _____ For what? ______________________
With injection? _____ Medication? _____ Other treatment? _____ How long? _____
Did you improve with treatment? ______________________
LIST ALL MEDICATIONS YOU ARE NOW TAKING: ______________________
Allergies to any medications (oral or injectable)? ______________________
Have you had any steroids (cortisone) in the past month? ______________________

DO YOU FEEL WE HAVE MISSED SOMETHING THAT IS PERTINENT TO YOUR SYMPTOMS? PLEASE LIST:

____

____

____

PLEASE RECHECK YOUR ANSWERS. IF YOU ARE SATISFIED THAT YOU HAVE ANSWERED TO THE FULLEST EXTENT, SEND THIS BACK TO THE OFFICE SO IT CAN BE EVALUATED. IF YOU HAVE NOT BEEN SEEN BY OUR DOCTOR, PLEASE BRING THIS QUESTIONNAIRE WITH YOU AT THE TIME OF YOUR INITIAL VISIT. THANK YOU.

Instructions for the Allergy Test

An appointment has been made on ________________ at ________ AM / PM

_____ Intradermal skin testing

_____ Skin testing for RAST correlation

1. In order to evaluate the allergy test accurately, certain medications should not be taken 48 hours before this test is performed. The medications include antihistamines and some tranquilizers.
2. Please complete the allergy questionnaire and mail it to the office if you have not already done so.
3. If you are running a fever or have an attack of asthma or hayfever, testing should be delayed.
4. If you, for the above or some other reason, cannot keep the appointment, please notify our office at least 2 days in advance; otherwise a charge may be made. If this date conflicts with previous plans, notify us immediately.
5. Do not change your diet before the test.
6. Make sure you eat breakfast before coming for a morning appointment, and lunch before an afternoon appointment.
7. Please wear short-sleeved or sleeveless apparel.
8. Bring a book, knitting, or something to pass the time between testings. The testing session may take 1 to 2½ hours, depending on the number of tests required. The tests may be completed in one session or it may take two, again depending on the number of tests required.

9. If an unusual symptom, such as sneezing, coughing, itching, hives, or asthma, occurs after the allergy testing, please contact our office.
10. If you are found to be allergic, your treatment will consist of periodic (weekly or twice weekly at the beginning) allergy injections that you may get at our office or at the doctor's office of your choice. However, we prefer that you come to our office so we can follow your allergic care more accurately, until your maintenance dose is established. At that time you may be taught to give your own injections or a member of your family may learn to administer them.

Letter to Patient's Family Physician

Dear Dr.

We have tested this patient for allergies and will be desensitizing the patient with antigen. This form of allergy is different from general allergy and is called skin endpoint titration. Through testing we have established the patient's degree of allergy to each individual inhalant and have mixed the antigen accordingly.

Our goal is to *relieve the patient's symptoms*. Please inquire at his injection how the patient's symptoms were after the previous injection and regulate the dosage accordingly. Continue to increase the dosage by 0.05-cc increments until you reach a dose that relieves that patient's symptoms for 1 week and repeat that dosage weekly. That will be the patient's maintenance dose.

If symptoms are not relieved by the time you reach the maximum dose of 0.5 cc, repeat that dose and indicate the patient's symptoms on his accompanying vial sheet. Have the patient call our office reporting no progress.

If the patient experiences arm reactions (a reaction being any itchy or red area the size of a fifty-cent piece, which lasts more than 24 hours) please drop back to the preceding dose. Hold that dose for 2 weeks and try to increase again. If you are unable to relieve symptoms because you cannot increase the dosage or antigen, please have your patient call our office.

Please return the accompanying vial sheet when there are two doses left in the vial so that the patient's treatment is not interrupted while we prepare a new vial.

Your communication on the vial sheet is important. Please indicate if and when there is symptom relief and how long that relief lasts.

Your help in treating this patient's allergies is greatly appreciated.

Sincerely,

North Hills Allergy Associates

Instructions for Administering Allergy Injections

Keep extracts in the refrigerator at all times, but do not freeze. Remove from the refrigerator about 15 minutes before administering injection(s) to allow the antigen to warm. Use allergy syringes with a 26-, 27-, or 27.5-gauge short shanked needle for administration. Disposable syringes should be used. Give injections at a 90° angle, straight in, in the fat back surface of the upper arm—not in the muscle!

A maximum dose of extract is 0.5 cc. Begin the patient on a dose of 0.05 cc of each vial, subcutaneously, not too shallow. Increase by 0.05 cc or by 0.1 cc each weekly injection as instructed, until the maximum dose is reached, *providing the patient does not have a reaction from a smaller dose*. The instructions are on the sheet provided with the vial.

Vial #1 should always be given in the right arm and Vial #2 should always be given in the left arm. If only one injection is given, alternate arms. The patient should remain in the doctor's office 10 to 20 minutes after injections. There may be local arm reactions that can be reported at the time of the next injection. Always ask the patient about reactions before drawing up antigens.

A patient's sensitivity to allergenic extracts change from time to time; therefore on some occasions a dose may be too large. In such a case, the patient may have sneezing or a watery, blocked nose and sometimes a clearing of mucus from the trachea or throat. Such a reaction would usually occur within 10 minutes after the injections are given and always within 6 to 8 hours. If this occurs, the patient may take a decongestant or antihistamine for relief. This reaction may be due to increased exposure to one of the patient's allergens and will usually not be repeated with increasing doses. Too low a dose may also provoke symptoms early in therapy.

Another sign of slightly too large a dose would be redness or soreness around the injection site. If the redness is the size of a fifty-cent piece or larger, and lasts more than 24 hours, drop to previous reaction-free dose and hold that dosage for two injections. Continue at the lower dosage only if the patient is symptom-free. If the patient is not symptom-free and is having no localized reactions, increase dosage again on the third injection. If a local arm reaction occurs again, call our office for further instructions. *Any reaction that lasts less than 24 hours* is usually due to skin sensitivity and the dose should not be lowered unless the reaction causes intolerable discomfort to the patient.

Stomach pain or cramps, diarrhea, sleepiness, headaches, fever, aching pains, etc. do not occur after these injections. If asthma is precipitated by an injection, *do not* give another injection until the patient is seen in this office.

We advance the patient's doses in order to stimulate the immune system. This should enable the patient to extend the time interval between injections and possibly to discontinue immunotherapy in the future.

Extracts are good for 2½ to 3 months if refrigerated. However, they do tend to lose some of their original potency. For this reason when the patient receives a new vial the first dose of that vial will usually be lowered on the new instruction sheet.

When it is apparent that there are only two doses left in the vial(s), please send back the sheet(s) as indicated so that the allergenic extracts may be renewed in time.

It is important to indicate on the vial sheet(s) the following:

- the dates and amounts of each injection.
- the patient's progress.
- any skin reactions.
- whether the vial should be mailed or left in our office to be picked up.

If you have any questions or comments concerning the patient's treatment or progress, please feel free to contact our office.

*If the patient is lax getting injections follow instructions below.

- Maintenance dose may be given up to 3 weeks.
- If between 3 and 6 weeks drop the dose by 0.2 and proceed weekly, increasing by 0.1 to maintenance.
- Patient may stretch injections every 2 to 3 weeks if symptom-free between injections.

Allergy Injection Techniques

It is important to know how to draw and inject your allergy medication properly. By learning to use the proper techniques, you or someone close to you can give quick, accurate injections, with a minimum of discomfort and inconvenience. It's easy if you follow these steps.

The most commonly used injection site is the fleshy area in back of your arm, when your doctor or someone else is giving the injection. Other possible sites—in the preferred order—are your midriff, abdomen or thigh. *Your doctor, however, will guide you in this important matter.*

Before the injection, be sure to have all of the necessary supplies ready: your bottle of allergy medication, alcohol swabs and your allergy syringe.

Note: Always inspect the allergy medication bottle before using it. Make sure the expiration date has not passed, and that the top of the bottle is in perfect condition, and undamaged.

You *must* use only allergy syringes, not insulin or tuberculin type.

This is the type of syringe you will receive from your pharmacy. Observe the markings and dosages shown along the syringe. Please make sure that you are giving the correct dose.

For safety, recap the needle and dispose of the needle and syringe so it cannot be used again.

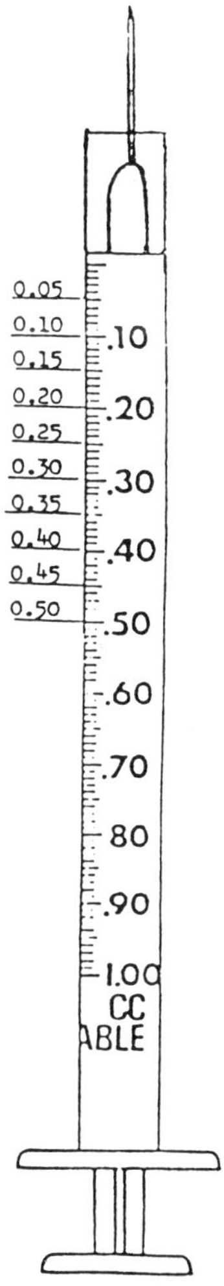

Drawing Allergy Medication*

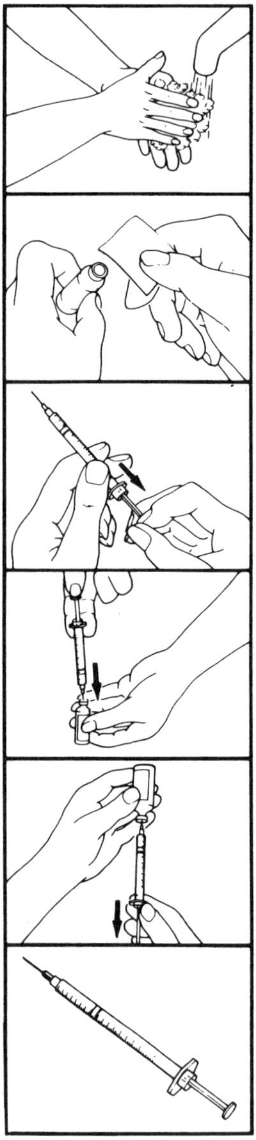

1. Before you begin, WASH YOUR HANDS.
2. Clean the rubber stopper on the allergy medication bottle with an alcohol swab.
3. Remove gray needle shield and white plunger cover on the B-D Allergy Syringe #5500. Draw air into the syringe by pulling out the plunger to the appropriate dose.
4. With the bottle standing upright, insert the needle into the rubber stopper on the bottle. Push in the plunger.
5. Turn the bottle and the syringe upside down. Slowly pull the plunger down, about .05 cc past your dose. If there are no air bubbles, push the top of the plunger tip up to the line which marks your exact dose.†
6. Remove the syringe from the bottle and carefully leave it on a flat surface until you are ready for injection. Avoid damage or contamination of the needle.

*This section is provided through the courtesy of Becton Dickinson and Company.

†NOTE: If air bubbles are in the syringe, remove them by tapping on the side of the syringe barrel. When the air bubbles go to the top of the syringe, push the plunger tip up to your exact dose.

Injecting Allergy Medication*

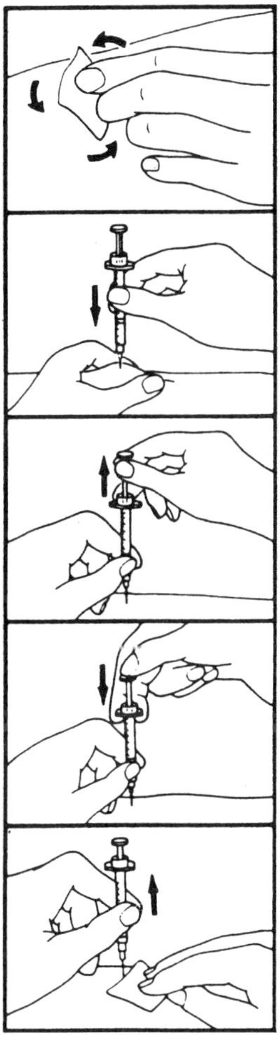

1. Clean the injection site with an alcohol swab, moving in a circular motion. Start from the center and move outward. Allow the alcohol to dry.
2. Carefully pick up the syringe. Pinch a two-inch fold of skin, and with one quick motion, inject the needle into the skin. The normal injection angle is between 45 degrees and 90 degrees, or straight in.
3. Release the pinched skin. While holding the barrel with one hand, pull back slightly on the plunger. Look for blood in the barrel. If there is blood, DO NOT INJECT THE ALLERGY MEDICATION. The needle is in a vessel. Simply pull the needle out of the injection site and start again with a new syringe and a new injection site.
4. If there is no blood, proceed with the injection by pushing the plunger down to inject the allergy medication.
5. When finished, pull the needle from the skin and gently hold an alcohol swab on the injection site. DO NOT MASSAGE THE AREA.
6. PLEASE DISPOSE OF SYRINGES PROPERLY
   Make the syringe unusable by carefully breaking off the needle. Drop the unusable syringe into an empty resealable container such as a coffee can, bleach bottle, or liquid detergent bottle.

KEEP THE CONTAINER OUT OF REACH OF CHILDREN.
When the container is full, seal the lid securely and deposit into the trash. Do not leave syringes intact so they can accidentally injure others. Contain them so they do not resurface in the wrong places. You may also return the used syringes to the office for disposal.

*This section is provided through the courtesy of Becton Dickinson and Company.

Appendix 3

Pollen Guide

The following guide is provided through the courtesy of Meridian Bio-Medical, Inc., Round Rock, Texas. The American Academy of Otolaryngic Allergy appreciates the cooperation of Meridian in sharing this information, which can be used as a point of departure for assessing regional aeroallergens of significance. Other factors to be considered by each individual are the results of local pollen surveys, the experience of others practicing in the area, and the clinician's continued observation of seasonal patterns of disease.

Richard L. Mabry, M.D., F.A.C.S., F.A.A.O.A.

Preface to the Pollen Guide

This reference has been prepared by Meridian Bio-Medical to provide botanical information for the physician interested in respiratory allergy. It contains a comprehensive list of important anemophilus (wind pollinated) plants indigenous to different regions within the Continental United States.

While there are thousands of seed bearing plants in the United States, only a small percentage are of medical importance. In order for the pollen of any plant to be important in pollinosis it must satisfy certain criteria as set forth in 1931 by A.A. Thommen in his five postulates.

Thommen's Postulates

1. The pollen must be wind borne (anemophilus). This requirement rules out showy flowered plants with sticky pollen which are insect pollinated.
2. The pollen must be produced in large quantities. This is a characteristic of wind pollinated plants.
3. The pollen must be sufficiently buoyant to be carried considerable distances. This would be those plants that produce pollen grains in the 15 to 58 micron range which are good floaters.
4. The plant producing the pollen must be widely and abundantly distributed.
5. The pollen must contain specific excitants or antigens for hypersensitivity.

It is important for the physician to keep these postulates in mind and acquaint himself with the flora of his area that satisfy these criteria.

The map and regional charts contained in this reference provide the physician with a convenient reference for plants that might be considered for diagnosis and therapy in various regions of the United States.

The regional charts indicate the time period that various plants usually pollinate within a given region. The actual pollinating dates may vary from year to year due to climatic conditions but will fall within the time frame indicated even though weather fronts and prevailing winds can affect the pollen season. It is also important to know that spring flowering plants bloom from South to North and that fall flowering plants bloom from North to South.

The second section represents a cross-index of synonymous names. Many plants have several common names and a few have new taxonomic names. This chart should serve to identify those plants that are known by several common and/or generic names.

The third section is a list of important hayfever plants arranged in phylogenetic order. This section provides the physician with information concerning closely related species; such information is important because antigen cross-reactivity may exist between members of the same family.

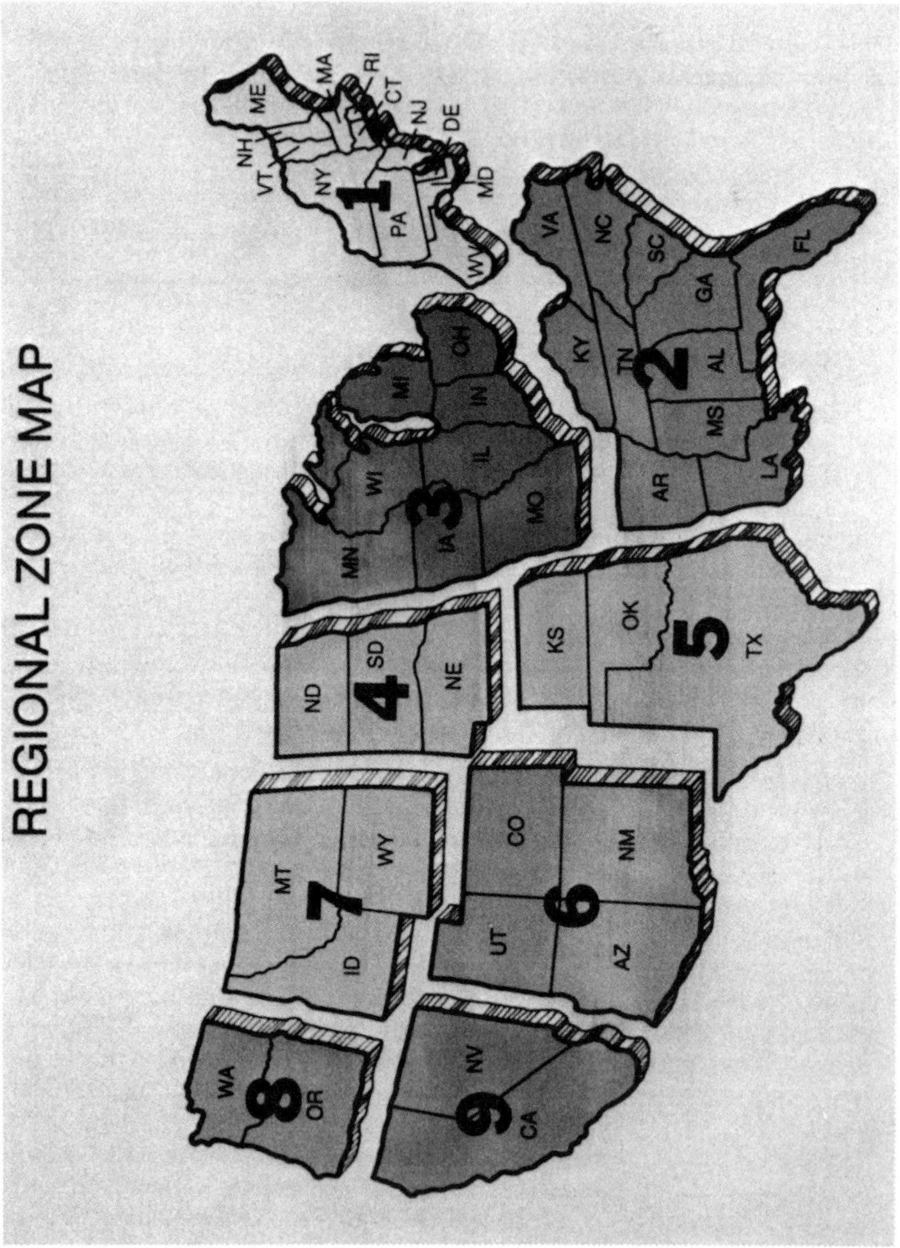
REGIONAL ZONE MAP
1
ME
NH
VT
MA
RI
CT
NJ
DE
MD
NY
PA
WV
2
VA
NC
SC
GA
FL
KY
TN
AL
MS
AR
LA
3
MI
OH
IN
WI
IL
MN
IA
MO
4
ND
SD
NE
5
KS
OK
TX
6
CO
NM
UT
AZ
7
MT
WY
ID
8
WA
OR
9
NV
CA

TREES

COMMON/SCIENTIFIC NAME	ZONE 1	ZONE 2	ZONE 3	ZONE 4	ZONE 5	ZONE 6	ZONE 7	ZONE 8	ZONE 9
ACACIA (Acacia spp.)		S Jan.-Feb.			S Jan.-Feb.	S Jan.-Feb.			W Jan.-Feb.
ALDER, RED (Alnus rubra)								W Feb.-Mar.	W Feb.-Mar.
ALDER, SMOOTH (Alnus rugosa)	Feb.-Mar.	Jan.-Feb.	Feb.-Mar.		E Jan.-Feb.				
ALDER, THINLEAF (Alnus tenuifolia)						Feb.-May	W Feb.-May	Feb.-May	Feb.-May
ALDER, WHITE (Alnus rhombifolia)								Feb.-Mar. •	W Feb.-Mar. •
ARBOR VITAE (Thuja orientalis)	Mar.-Apr.	Mar.-Apr.	Mar.-Apr.						
ASH, ARIZONA (Fraxinus velutina)					S Mar.-Apr. •	SW Mar.-Apr. •			S Mar.-Apr. •
ASH, OREGON (Fraxinus oregona)								Mar.-Apr. •	Mar.-Apr. •
ASH, GREEN (Fraxinus pennsylvanica)	Apr.-May •	Mar.-May •	Apr.-May •	Apr-May	E Mar.-Apr. •		E Apr.-May		
ASH, WHITE (Fraxinus americana)	Apr.-May •	Mar.-May •	S Apr.-May •		E Mar.-Apr. •				
ASPEN, QUAKING (Populus tremuloides)	Apr.-May		Apr.-May			Apr.-May •	Apr.-May •	Apr.-May •	Apr.-May •
BACCHARIS (Baccharis spp.) †		S Sep.-Oct.			S Sep.-Oct.	S Sep.-Oct.			S Sep.-Oct.
BEECH, AMERICAN (Fagus grandifolia)	Apr.-May •	Apr.-May •	E Apr.-May •						
BIRCH, PAPER (Betula papyrifera)	Apr.-Jun. •		N Apr.-Jun. •				N Apr.-Jun. •	N Apr.-Jun. •	
BIRCH, RED (Betula nigra) †	Apr.-Jun. •	Apr.-May	Apr.-Jun. •		E Apr.-May				
BIRCH, RIVER (Betula nigra) †	Apr.-Jun. •	Apr.-May	Apr.-Jun. •		E Apr.-May				
BIRCH, SWEET (Betula lenta)	Apr.-May •	N Apr.-May	E Apr.-May •						
BIRCH, WHITE (Betula populifolia)	Apr.-Jun. •		N Apr.-Jun. •						
BIRCH, YELLOW (Betula alleghaniensis)	Apr.-May •	Apr.-May	Apr.-May •						

TREES (continued)

COMMON/SCIENTIFIC NAME	ZONE 1	ZONE 2	ZONE 3	ZONE 4	ZONE 5	ZONE 6	ZONE 7	ZONE 8	ZONE 9
BOX ELDER (Acer negundo)	Apr.-May •	Mar.-May •	Apr.-May •	Apr.-May •	Mar.-Apr. •	Mar.-May •	May •		Mar.-Apr. •
CEDAR, DEODARA (Cedrus deodara)									Jan.-Feb.
CEDAR, INCENSE (Libocedrus decurrens)									Jan.-Feb.
CEDAR, PINCHOT (Juniperus pinchotii) †					Sep.-Nov. •	S Sep.-Nov. •			
CEDAR, MOUNTAIN (Juniperus sabinoides)		NW Dec.-Jan. •	SW Dec.-Jan. •		Dec.-Jan. •				
CEDAR, RED (Juniperus virginiana)	Mar.-Apr.	Feb.-Apr.	Mar.-Apr.	E Mar.-Apr.	E Feb.-Mar.				
CHINESE TALLOW (Sapium sebiferum)		S May-Jun.			S May-Jun.				
COTTONWOOD, ARIZONA (Populus fremontii) †						W Mar.-Apr. •			Mar.-Apr. •
COTTONWOOD, BLACK (Populus trichocarpa)							W May-Jun. •	Apr.-May •	Apr.-May •
COTTONWOOD, COMMON (Populus deltoides) †		Mar.-Apr. •	Mar.-Apr. •	SE Apr. •	E Mar.-Apr. •				
COTTONWOOD, EASTERN (Populus deltoides) †		Mar.-Apr. •	Mar.-Apr. •	SE Apr. •	E Mar.-Apr. •				
COTTONWOOD, RIO GRANDE (Populus wislizenii)						Mar.-Apr.			
COTTONWOOD, WESTERN (Populus sargentii)				Apr.-May •	Mar.-Apr. •	NE Apr. •	E Apr.-May •		
CYPRESS, ARIZONA (Cupressus arizonica)					SW Jan.-Feb.	S Jan.-Feb. •			S Jan.-Feb. •
CYPRESS, BALD (Taxodium distichum)		Jan.-Feb.			Jan.-Feb.				
CYPRESS, MONTEREY (Cupressus macrocarpa)									W Jan.-Feb. •
DATE (Phoenix dactylifera)		Jan-Feb.							Jan.-Feb.
DATE, CANARY (Phoenix canariensis)		S Jan.-Feb.							S Jan.-Feb.
ELM, AMERICAN (Ulmus americana)	Feb.-Apr. •	Jan.-Mar. •	Feb.-Apr. •	Mar.-Apr. •	Jan.-Mar. •				

† This plant is also known by another name; consult Synonomous Names Cross Reference for other name(s).
N, S, E, W Indicates this plant is found in the Northern, Southern, Eastern, or Western region of that particular zone.
• Primary allergic significance due to either volume of pollen produced, potency of pollen produced, or a combination of the two.

TREES (continued)

	COMMON/SCIENTIFIC NAME	ZONE 1	ZONE 2	ZONE 3	ZONE 4	ZONE 5	ZONE 6	ZONE 7	ZONE 8	ZONE 9
TREES	ELM, CEDAR (Ulmus crassifolia) †		W Aug.-Sep. •			E Aug.-Sep. •				
	ELM, CHINESE (Ulmus pumila)			W Feb.-Apr. •	Feb.-Apr. •	Jan.-Mar. •	Jan.-Apr. •	Mar.-Apr. •	Feb.-Apr. •	Jan.-Apr. •
	ELM, FALL BLOOMING (Ulmus crassifolia) †		W Aug.-Sep. •			E Aug.-Sep. •				
	ELM, FALL BLOOMING (Ulmus parvifolia)		Aug.-Sep.			Aug.-Sep.	Aug.-Sep.			Aug.-Sep. •
	EUCALYPTUS spp.									Nov.-Jan.
	GROUNDSEL TREE (Baccharis spp.) †		S Sep.-Oct.			S Sep.-Oct.	S Sep.-Oct.			S Sep.-Oct.
	HACKBERRY (Celtis occidentalis)	Mar.-Apr.	Feb.-Apr.	Feb.-Apr.	Mar.-Apr.	Feb.-Apr.				
	HAZELNUT (Corylus americana)	Feb.-Apr.	Feb.-Apr.	Feb.-Apr.						
	HAZELNUT, CALIF. (Corylus californica)								Feb.-Apr.	Feb.-Apr.
	HICKORY, BITTERNUT (Carya cordiformis)	Apr.-May •	N Apr.-May •	Apr.-May •		E Apr.-May •				
	HICKORY, PIGNUT (Carya glabra)	S May-Jun. •	Mar.-May •	Apr.-May •						
	HICKORY, SHAGBARK (Carya ovata)	Apr.-May •	N Apr.-May •	S Apr.-May •						
	HICKORY, SHELLBARK (Carya laciniosa)		N Apr.-May •	S Apr.-Jun. •						
	HICKORY, WHITE (Carya tomentosa)	Apr.-Jun. •	Apr.-May •	Apr.-May •		E Apr.-May •				
	HORNBEAM (Carpinus caroliniana)	Apr.-May	Mar.-May	Apr.-May		E Mar.-Apr.				
	IRONWOOD (Ostrya virginiana)	Apr.-May	N Mar.-May	Apr.-Jun.	E Apr.-May	E Mar.-Apr.				
	JUNIPER, ALLIGATOR (Juniperus deppeana)					W Feb.-Apr.	Mar.-Apr. •			
	JUNIPER, ONESEED (Juniperus monosperma)					W Mar.-Apr.	Mar.-Apr. •			
	JUNIPER, REDBERRY (Juniperus pinchotii) †					Sep.-Nov. •	S Sep.-Nov. •			

TREES (continued)

COMMON/SCIENTIFIC NAME	ZONE 1	ZONE 2	ZONE 3	ZONE 4	ZONE 5	ZONE 6	ZONE 7	ZONE 8	ZONE 9
JUNIPER, ROCKY MTN. (Juniperus scopulorum)						Feb.-Apr. •	Mar.-Apr. •	E Mar.-Apr. •	E Mar.-Apr. •
JUNIPER, UTAH (Juniperus osteosperma)						Mar.-Apr. •	Mar.-Apr. •		E Mar.-Apr. •
JUNIPER, WESTERN (Juniperus occidentalis)									Dec.-Feb. •
LIGUSTRUM (Ligustrum spp.) †	Apr.-Jun.	Apr.-Jun.	May-Jun.	May-Jun.	Apr.-Jun. •	Apr.-Jun. •	Apr.-Jun.	May-Jun.	Apr.-Jun. •
LINDEN, BASSWOOD (Tilia spp.)	Jun.-Jul.	N Jun.-Jul.	Jun.-Jul.						
MAPLE, COAST (Acer macrophyllum)								W Apr.-May	W Apr.-May
MAPLE, HARD (Acer saccharum) †	Apr.-May •	N Apr.-May •	Apr.-May •						
MAPLE, RED (Acer rubrum)	Feb.-May •	Feb.-Mar. •	Feb.-May •		E Feb.-Mar.				
MAPLE, SILVER (Acer saccharinum) †	Feb.-Apr. •	Feb.-Mar. •	Feb.-Apr. •		Feb.-Mar. •				
MAPLE, SOFT (Acer saccharinum) †	Feb.-Apr. •	Feb.-Mar. •	Feb.-Apr. •		Feb.-Mar. •				
MAPLE, SUGAR (Acer saccharum) †	Apr.-May •	N Apr.-May •	Apr.-May •						
MESQUITE (Prosopis spp.)					S Apr.-Jun. •	S Apr.-Jun. •			S Apr.-Jun. •
MULBERRY, PAPER (Broussonetia papyrifera)	S May-Jun.	Apr.-May	May-Jun.		E Apr.-May				
MULBERRY, RED (Morus rubra)	May-Jun.	Apr.-May	Apr.-Jun.		E Apr.-May	S Apr.-May			S Apr.-May
MULBERRY, WHITE (Morus alba)	May-Jun.	Apr.-May	Apr.-Jun.		E Apr.-May	S Mar.-Apr.			S Mar.-Apr.
OAK, BLACK (Quercus velutina)	Apr.-Jun. •	Apr.-May •	Apr.-May •		E Apr.-May •				
OAK, BLACKJACK (Quercus marilandica)		Apr.-May •	SW Apr.-May		E Apr.-May •				
OAK, BLUE (Quercus douglasii)									W Mar.-Apr. •
OAK, BUR (Quercus macrocarpa)		NW Apr.-May •	May-Jun. •	May-Jun. •	Apr.-May •				

† This plant is also known by another name; consult Synonomous Names Cross Reference for other name(s).

N, S, E, W Indicates this plant is found in the Northern, Southern, Eastern, or Western region of that particular zone.

• Primary allergic significance due to either volume of pollen produced, potency of pollen produced, or a combination of the two.

TREES (continued)

	COMMON/SCIENTIFIC NAME	ZONE 1	ZONE 2	ZONE 3	ZONE 4	ZONE 5	ZONE 6	ZONE 7	ZONE 8	ZONE 9
TREES	OAK, CALIFORNIA BLACK (Quercus kellogii)									W Mar.-Apr. •
	OAK, CALIFORNIA LIVE (Quercus agrifolia)									W Mar.-Apr. •
	OAK, CALIFORNIA SCRUB (Quercus dumosa)									W Mar.-Apr. •
	OAK, CALIFORNIA WHITE (Quercus lobata)									W Mar.-Apr. •
	OAK, CANYON LIVE (Quercus chrysolepsis)									W Mar.-Apr. •
	OAK, GAMBEL'S (Quercus gambelii)						Apr.-Jun. •	S May-Jun. •		
	OAK, LIVE (Quercus virginiana)		S Mar.-Apr. •			S Mar.-Apr. •				
	OAK, PIN (Quercus palustris)	S Apr.-May •	N Apr.-May	Apr.-May •		E Apr.-May				
	OAK, POST (Quercus stellata)	S Apr.-May •	Mar.-May •	S Mar.-Apr. •		Mar.-Apr. •				
	OAK, RED (Quercus rubra)	Apr.-May •	N Mar.-May	Apr.-May •		E Apr.-May •				
	OAK, SPANISH (Quercus coccinea)	S Apr.-May	N Apr.-May	S Apr.-May						
	OAK, SOUTHERN RED (Quercus falcata)	S Apr.-May	Apr.-May •			E Apr.-May •				
	OAK, WATER (Quercus nigra)		Mar.-May •							
	OAK, WHITE (Quercus alba)	Apr.-May •	Mar.-May •	Apr.-May •		SE Mar.-May •				
	OAK, WILLOW (Quercus phellos)	SE Apr.-May	Mar.-May •							
	OLIVE (Olea europaea)						S Apr.-May •			S Apr.-May •
	PECAN (Carya illinoensis) †		W Apr.-May	S Apr.-May •		E Apr.-May •				
	PEPPERTREE (Schinus molle)						S Jun.-Jul.			Jun.-Jul.
	PINE, AUSTRIAN (Pinus nigra)	Apr.-Jun.	Apr.-Jun.	Apr.-Jun.	May-Jun.	Apr.-May	Apr.-May	May-Jun.	Apr.-Jun.	Apr.-May

TREES (continued)

COMMON/SCIENTIFIC NAME	ZONE 1	ZONE 2	ZONE 3	ZONE 4	ZONE 5	ZONE 6	ZONE 7	ZONE 8	ZONE 9
PINE, LOBLOLLY (Pinus taeda)		Apr.-May			SE Apr.-May				
PINE, LODGEPOLE (Pinus contorta)							May-Jul.	May-Jul.	May-Jul.
PINE, LONGLEAF (Pinus palustris)		Feb.-Apr.			Mar.-Apr.				
PINE, PONDEROSA (Pinus ponderosa)				W May-Jun.		Apr.-Jun.	May-Jun.	May-Jun.	Apr.-Jun.
PINE, RED (Pinus resinosa)	May-Jun.		May-Jun.						
PINE, SCOTCH (Pinus sylvestris)	Apr.-Jun.		Apr.-Jun.		Apr.-May				
PINE, SHORTLEAF (Pinus echinata)	S Apr.-May	Mar.-May	S Apr.-May		E Mar.-May				
PINE, SLASH (Pinus elliotti)		S Jan.-Mar.							
PINE, WHITE (Pinus strobus)	Jun.-Jul.	NE May-Jun.	NE Jun.-Jul.						
PLANETREE, LONDON (Platanus acerifolia)	May-Jun.	May-Jun.							Apr.-May
POPLAR, FREMONT (Populus fremontii) †						W Mar.-Apr. •			Mar.-Apr. •
POPLAR, LOMBARDY (Populus nigra italica)	Mar.-Apr.	Feb.-Mar.	Mar.-Apr.	Mar.-Apr.	Feb.-Mar.	Feb.-Mar.	Mar.-May	Mar.-May	Feb.-Apr.
POPLAR, WHITE (Populus alba)	Mar.-Apr.	Feb.-Apr.	S Mar.-Apr.	S Mar.-Apr.	Feb.-Apr.	Feb.-Mar.	S Mar.-May	Mar.-May	Feb.-Apr.
PRIVET (Ligustrum spp.) †	Apr.-Jun.	Apr.-Jun.	May-Jun.	May-Jun.	Apr.-Jun. •	Apr.-Jun. •	Apr.-Jun.	May-Jun.	Apr.-Jun. •
SALT CEDAR (Tamarix gallica)		May-Sep.			May-Sep.	May-Sep.		S May-Sep.	May-Sep.
SPRUCE, BLUE (Picea pungens)						Apr.-May	Apr.-May		
SPRUCE, RED (Picea rubens)	Apr.-May	NE Apr.-May							
SWEETGUM (Liquidambar styraciflua)	S Apr.-May	Mar.-May	S Apr.-May		E Mar.-May	S Mar.-Apr.			S Mar.-Apr.
SYCAMORE (Platanus occidentalis)	Apr.-May •	Mar.-May •	Apr.-May •		Mar.-May •				Apr.-May

† This plant is also known by another name; consult Synonomous Names Cross Reference for other name(s).

N, S, E, W Indicates this plant is found in the Northern, Southern, Eastern, or Western region of that particular zone.

• Primary allergic significance due to either volume of pollen produced, potency of pollen produced, or a combination of the two.

TREES (continued)

TREES

COMMON/SCIENTIFIC NAME	ZONE 1	ZONE 2	ZONE 3	ZONE 4	ZONE 5	ZONE 6	ZONE 7	ZONE 8	ZONE 9
SYCAMORE, CALIFORNIA (Platanus racemosa)								S Feb.-Apr. •	Feb.-Apr. •
TREE-OF-HEAVEN (Ailanthus altissima)	Jun.-Jul.	May-Jul.	May-Jul.	Jun.-Jul.	May-Jul.	May-Jul.	Jun.-Jul.	Jun.-Jul.	May-Jul.
WALNUT, BLACK (Juglans nigra)	May-Jun. •	Apr.-Jun. •	May-Jun. •	E May-Jun.	Apr.-Jun. •				
WALNUT, CALIF. BLACK (Juglans californica)									Mar.-Apr. •
WALNUT, ENGLISH (Juglans regia)								S Apr.-May •	Mar.-Apr. •
WALNUT, MEXICAN (Juglans rupestris)								S Mar.-May •	
WHITE FIR (Abies grandis)							W May-Jun.	Apr.-May	Apr.-May
WILLOW, BLACK (Salix nigra)	Apr.-Jun.	Feb.-May	Apr.-Jun.	Apr.-Jun.	Feb.-Jun.	Feb.-Jun.	May-Jun.	Apr.-Jun.	Feb.-Jun.

WEEDS

COMMON/SCIENTIFIC NAME	ZONE 1	ZONE 2	ZONE 3	ZONE 4	ZONE 5	ZONE 6	ZONE 7	ZONE 8	ZONE 9
ALLSCALE (Atriplex polycarpa)						W Jul.-Oct.			Jul.-Oct.
AMARANTH, GREEN (Amaranthus hybridus)	Jul.-Aug. •	Jul.-Oct.	S Jul.-Sep. •	Jul.-Sep. •	Jul.-Oct.	Jul.-Oct.			Jul.-Oct. •
BASSIA (Bassia hyssopifolia)	Jul.-Oct.							Jul.-Oct.	W Jul.-Oct.
BEACH SANDBUR (Franseria bipinnitifida)								W Mar.-Nov.	W Mar.-Nov.
BEACHWEED, SILVER (Franseria chamissonis)								Jul.-Nov.	Jul.-Nov.
BROOMWEED (Gutierrezia dracunculoides)			S Jul.-Oct.		Jul.-Oct.	Jul.-Oct.			
BURNING BUSH (Kochia scoparia) †				Jul.-Sep. •	Jul.-Oct. •	Jul.-Oct. •	Jul.-Sep. •	Jul.-Aug. •	Jul.-Oct. •
BURROBRUSH (Hymenoclea monogyra)						Aug.-Nov.			Aug.-Nov.
BURROBRUSH, WHITE (Hymenoclea salsola)						Mar.-Apr.			Mar.-Apr.
CARELESSWEED (Amaranthus palmeri) †	Jul.-Oct.	W Jul.-Oct. •	S Jul.-Oct. •		Jul.-Oct. •	S Jul.-Oct. •			S Jun.-Oct.
COCKLEBUR (Xanthium commune) †	Aug.-Sep. •	Aug.-Oct. •	Aug.-Sep. •	Aug.-Sep. •	Aug.-Oct. •	Aug.-Oct. •	Jul.-Sep. •	Jul.-Sep.	Aug.-Oct. •
DOCK, BITTER (Rumex obtusifolia)	May-Jun.	Apr.-May	May-Jun.	May-Jun.	Apr.-May	Apr.-May	May-Jun.	May-Jun.	Apr.-Jun.
DOCK, SOUR (Rumex acetosella) †	Apr.-May •	Apr.-May •	Apr.-Jun. •	May-Jun. •	Apr.-May •	Apr.-May	May-Jun. •	May-Jun. •	Apr.-May •
DOCK, TALL (Rumex altissimus)	Apr.-May	Apr.-May	Apr.-May		Apr.-May	Apr.-Jun.			
DOCK, WHITE (Rumex mexicanus)	Apr.-May		Apr.-May	Apr.-May	Apr.-May	Apr.-May	Apr.-May		
DOCK, YELLOW (Rumex crispus)	Apr.-May	Apr.-May	Apr.-May	Apr.-May	Apr.-May	Apr.-May	Apr.-May	Apr.-May	Apr.-May
FIREBUSH (Kochia scoparia) †				Jul-Sep. •	Jul.-Oct. •	Jul.-Oct. •	Jul.-Sep. •	Jul.-Aug. •	Jul.-Oct. •
GOLDENROD (Solidago spp.)	Aug.-Sep.	Aug.-Oct.	Aug.-Sep.	Aug.-Sep.	Aug.-Oct.	Aug.-Oct.	Aug.-Sep.	Aug.-Sep.	Aug.-Oct.
GREASEWOOD (Sarcobatus vermiculatus)					W Jun.-Jul.	Jun.-Jul. •	Jun.-Jul. •	E Jun.-Jul.	E Jun.-Jul. •

† This plant is also known by another name; consult Synonomous Names Cross Reference for other name(s).
N, S, E, W Indicates this plant is found in the Northern, Southern, Eastern, or Western region of that particular zone.
• Primary allergic significance due to either volume of pollen produced, potency of pollen produced, or a combination of the two.

WEEDS (continued)

WEEDS: COMMON/SCIENTIFIC NAME	ZONE 1	ZONE 2	ZONE 3	ZONE 4	ZONE 5	ZONE 6	ZONE 7	ZONE 8	ZONE 9
INDIAN HAIR TONIC (Artemisia dracunculus) †			Jul.-Aug.	Jul.-Aug.	Jul.-Aug.	Jul.-Aug. •			Jul.-Aug.
IODINE BUSH (Allenrolfea occidentalis)					Jun.-Jul.	Jun.-Aug.			Jun.-Aug.
JERUSALEM OAK (Chenopodium botrys)	Jul.-Aug.	Jul.-Aug.	Jul.-Aug.	Jun.-Jul.	Jul.-Aug.	Jun.-Oct.	Jun.-Jul.	Jun.-Jul.	Jul.-Sep.
KOCHIA (Kochia scoparia) †				Jul.-Sep. •	Jul.-Oct. •	Jul.-Oct. •	Jul.-Sep. •	Jul.-Aug. •	Jul.-Oct. •
LAMB'S QUARTERS (Chenopodium album)	Aug.-Sep. •	Aug.-Sep. •	Aug.-Sep. •	Aug.-Sep. •	Sep.-Oct. •	Sep.-Oct. •	Aug.-Sep. •	Aug.-Sep. •	Aug.-Oct. •
LENSCALE (Atriplex lentiformis)						Aug.-Sep.			Aug.-Sep. •
MARSH ELDER, BURWEED (Iva xanthifolia)			Aug.-Sep. •	Aug.-Sep. •	Sep.-Oct. •	Aug.-Oct. •	Aug.-Sep. •	Aug.-Sep. •	
MARSH ELDER, NARROWLEAF (Iva angustifolia)		W Aug.-Sep.			E Aug.-Sep. •				
MARSH ELDER, ROUGH (Iva ciliata) †		Aug.-Oct.	Aug.-Sep. •		Aug.-Oct. •	S Aug.-Sep. •			
MARSH ELDER, TRUE (Iva ciliata) †		Aug.-Oct.	Aug.-Sep. •		Aug.-Oct. •	Aug.-Sep. •			
MEXICAN FIREBUSH (Kochia scoparia) †				Jul.-Sep. •	Jul.-Oct. •	Jul.-Oct. •	Jul.-Sep. •	Jul.-Aug. •	Jul.-Oct. •
MEXICAN TEA (Chenopodium ambrosioides)	Aug.-Sep.	Aug.-Oct.	Aug.-Sep.		Aug.-Oct.	Aug.-Oct.			Aug.-Oct.
MUGWORT, CALIF. (Artemisia heterophylla)									Sep.-Oct. •
MUGWORT, COMMON (Artemisia vulgaris)	Aug.-Sep.	E Sep.-Oct.	E Aug.-Sep.						
MUGWORT, DARK-LEAVED (Artemisia ludoviciana)		W Sep.-Oct.	S Sep.-Oct.		Sep.-Oct. •	Sep.-Oct. •	S Sep.		
NETTLE (Urtica spp.)	Jul.-Aug.	Aug.-Sep.	Jul.-Aug.	Jul.-Aug.	Aug.-Sep.	Jul.-Sep.	Jul.-Aug.	Jul.-Aug.	Jul.-Sep.
PALMER'S AMARANTH (Amaranthus palmerii) †	Jul.-Oct.	W Jul.-Oct. •	S Jul.-Oct. •		Jul.-Oct. •	S Jul.-Oct. •			S Jun.-Oct.
PIGWEED, SPINY (Amaranthus spinosus)	Jun.-Aug. •	Jun.-Aug. •	Jun.-Aug. •		Jun.-Aug. •				
PIGWEED, ROUGH (Amaranthus retroflexus) †	Jul.-Sep. •	Jul.-Oct. •	Jul.-Oct. •	Jul.-Sep. •	Jul.-Oct. •	Jul.-Oct. •	Jul.-Sep. •	Jul.-Sep. •	Jul.-Oct. •

WEEDS (continued)

	COMMON/SCIENTIFIC NAME	ZONE 1	ZONE 2	ZONE 3	ZONE 4	ZONE 5	ZONE 6	ZONE 7	ZONE 8	ZONE 9
WEEDS	PIGWEED, REDROOT (Amaranthus retroflexus) †	Jul.-Sep. •	Jul.-Oct. •	Jul.-Sep. •	Jul.-Sep. •	Jul.-Oct. •	Jul.-Oct. •	Jul.-Sep. •	Jul.-Sep. •	Jul.-Oct. •
	PLANTAIN, ENGLISH (Plantago lanceolata)	May-Jul. •	Apr.-Jun. •	May-Jul. •	Jun.-Jul. •	Apr.-Jul. •	Apr.-Aug. •	Jun.-Jul.•	May-Jul. •	Apr.-Aug. •
	POVERTYWEED (Iva axillaris)						May-Jul. •	Jun.-Jul. •	May-Jul. •	May-Jul. •
	PRIONOPSIS (Haplopappus ciliatus)			SW Aug.-Sep.		Aug.-Sep.	E Aug.-Sep.			
	RABBIT BUSH (Franseria deltoidea)						S Mar.-Apr. •			
	RAGWEED, CANYON (Franseria ambrosioides)						SE Mar.-May •			S Mar.-May
	RAGWEED, DESERT (Franseria dumosa)						W Mar.-Apr. •			SE Mar.-Apr. •
	RAGWEED, FALSE (Franseria acanthicarpa)					W Aug.-Sep. •	Aug.-Sep. •	Aug.-Sep. •	Aug.-Sep. •	Aug.-Sep. •
	RAGWEED, GIANT (Ambrosia trifida)	Aug.-Sep. •	Aug.-Oct. •	Aug.-Sep. •	Aug.-Sep. •	Aug.-Oct. •	E Aug.-Sep. •	E Aug.-Sep.		Aug.-Oct.
	RAGWEED, SHORT (Ambrosia artemisiifolia) †	Aug.-Sep. •	Aug.-Oct. •	Aug.-Sep. •	Aug.-Sep. •	Aug.-Oct. •	E Aug.-Sep.	E Aug.-Sep.		Aug.-Oct.
	RAGWEED, SILVER (Dicoria canescens)						W Aug.-Sep.			SE Aug.-Sep.
	RAGWEED, SLENDER (Franseria tenuifolia)					W Aug.-Oct. •	Aug.-Oct. •			S Aug.-Oct.
	RAGWEED, SOUTHERN (Ambrosia bidentata)		W Aug.-Sep.	S Aug.-Sep. •		Aug.-Sep. •				
	RAGWEED, WESTERN (Ambrosia coronopifolia) †			W Aug.-Sep. •	Aug.-Sep. •	Aug.-Oct. •	Aug.-Oct. •	Aug.-Sep. •		Aug.-Oct. •
	RAGWEED, WESTERN GIANT (Ambrosia aptera)			SW Aug.-Sep.	S Aug.-Sep.	Aug.-Oct. •	Aug.-Oct. •			
	RAGWEED, WOOLLY (Franseria tomentosa)					W Aug.-Sep.	E Aug.-Sep.			
	RUSSIAN THISTLE (Salsola kali tenuifolia) †				Jul.-Sep. •	Jul.-Sep. •	Jul.-Sep. •	Jul.-Aug. •	Jul.-Aug. •	E Jul.-Sep. •
	SAGE, DRAGON (Artemisia dracunculus) †			Jul.-Aug.	Jul.-Aug.	Jul.-Aug.	Jul.-Aug. •			Jul.-Aug.
	SAGE, CARPET (Artemisia frigida) †			NW Aug.-Sep.	NW Aug.-Sep.		Aug.-Oct. •	Aug.-Sep. •		NE Aug.-Sep.

† This plant is also known by another name; consult Synonomous Names Cross Reference for other name(s).
N, S, E, W Indicates this plant is found in the Northern, Southern, Eastern, or Western region of that particular zone.
• Primary allergic significance due to either volume of pollen produced, potency of pollen produced, or a combination of the two.

WEEDS (continued)

WEEDS COMMON/SCIENTIFIC NAME	ZONE 1	ZONE 2	ZONE 3	ZONE 4	ZONE 5	ZONE 6	ZONE 7	ZONE 8	ZONE 9
SAGE, GREEN (Artemisia dracunuculus) †			Jul.-Aug.	Jul.-Aug.	Jul.-Aug.	Jul.-Aug. •			Jul.-Aug.
SAGEBRUSH, COMMON (Artemisia tridentata)						Sep.-Oct. •	Aug.-Sep. •	Aug.-Sep. •	Sep.-Oct. •
SAGEBRUSH, COAST (Artemisia californica)									SW Sep.-Oct. •
SAGE, PASTURE (Artemisia frigida) †			NW Aug.-Sep.	NW Aug.-Sep.		Aug.-Oct. •	Aug.-Sep. •		NE Aug.-Sep.
SAGE, PRAIRIE (Artemisia gnaphalodes)			W Sep.-Oct.	Sep.-Oct.	Sep.-Oct. •	Sep.-Oct. •	Aug.-Sep.	E Aug.-Sep.	E Sep.-Oct.
SAGEBRUSH, SAND (Artemisia filifolia)				SW Aug.-Sep. •	W Aug.-Sep. •	Aug.-Oct. •	SE Aug.-Sep.		NE Aug.-Sep.
SALTBUSH, ANNUAL (Atriplex wrightii)						S Jul.-Aug.			
SALTBUSH, COAST (Atriplex breweri)									S Jul.-Aug.
SEA BLITE (Suaeda spp.)	E Jul.-Aug.	SE Jul.-Aug.		W Jul.-Aug.	SW Jul.-Aug.	Jul.-Sep.	Jul.-Aug.	Jul.-Aug.	Jul.-Sep.
SHADSCALE (Atriplex confertifolia)						May-Jun. •	May-Jun. •	SE May-Jun.	May-Jun.
SHEEP SORREL (Rumex acetosella) †	Apr.-May •	Apr.-May •	Apr.-Jun. •	May-Jun. •	Apr.-May •	Apr.-May	May-Jun. •	May-Jun. •	Apr.-May •
SILVERSCALE (Atriplex argentea)				Jul.-Aug.	Jul.-Aug.	Jun.-Aug.	Jul.-Aug.	SE Jul.-Aug.	NE Jun.-Aug.
SPEARSCALE (Atriplex patula)	Jul.-Sep.	Jul.-Oct.	Jul.-Sep.	Jul.-Aug.	Jul.-Oct.	Jul.-Oct.	Jul.-Aug.	Jul.-Aug.	Jul.-Oct.
TUMBLEWEED (Salsola kali tenuifolia) †				Jul.-Sep. •	Jul.-Sep. •	Jul.-Sep. •	Jul.-Aug. •	Jul.-Aug. •	E Jul.-Sep. •
WESTERN WATER HEMP (Acnida tamariscina)		W Jul.-Sep.	SW Jul.-Sep.	SE Jul.-Aug. •	Jul.-Oct. •	E Jul.-Oct. •			
WILD RHUBARB (Rumex hymenocephalus)						Mar.-May			Mar.-May
WINGSCALE (Atriplex canescens)				W Jun.-Jul.	W Jun.-Jul.	Jun.-Jul. •	Jun.-Jul. •	Jun.-Jul. •	Jun.-Jul. •
WINTER FAT (Eurotia lanata)				W Jun.-Jul.	W Jun.-Jul.	Jun.-Jul.	Jun.-Jul.	Jun.-Jul.	Jun.-Jul.
WORMWOOD, ANNUAL (Artemisia annua)	Aug.-Sep. •	Aug.-Oct. •	Aug.-Sep.	SE Aug.-Sep.	NE Aug.-Sep.				

WEEDS (continued)

COMMON/SCIENTIFIC NAME	ZONE 1	ZONE 2	ZONE 3	ZONE 4	ZONE 5	ZONE 6	ZONE 7	ZONE 8	ZONE 9
WORMWOOD, BIENNIAL (Artemisia biennis)	Aug.-Sep.		Aug.-Sep.	Aug.-Sep.		Aug.-Oct.	Aug.-Sep.	Aug.-Sep.	Aug.-Oct.
WORMWOOD, COMMON (Artemisia absinthium)	Aug.-Sep. •		Aug.-Sep.	N Aug.-Sep. •			Aug. •	Aug. •	
WORMWOOD, SAGEWORT (Artemisia campestris)	Aug.-Sep.	E Aug.-Sep.	Aug.-Sep.	Aug.-Sep.		Aug.-Sep.	Aug.-Sep.	Aug.-Sep.	

WEEDS

† This plant is also known by another name; consult Synonomous Names Cross Reference for other name(s).

N, S, E, W Indicates this plant is found in the Northern, Southern, Eastern, or Western region of that particular zone.

• Primary allergic significance due to either volume of pollen produced, potency of pollen produced, or a combination of the two.

GRASSES

COMMON/SCIENTIFIC NAME	ZONE 1	ZONE 2	ZONE 3	ZONE 4	ZONE 5	ZONE 6	ZONE 7	ZONE 8	ZONE 9
BAHIA (Paspalum notatum)		S May-Oct.			SE May-Oct.				
BERMUDA GRASS (Cynodon dactylon)	S Jun.-Sep. •	May-Sep. •	S Jun.-Sep. •		May-Oct. •	May-Oct. •			May-Oct. •
BLUEGRASS, ANNUAL (Poa annua)	Feb.-Jun.	Jan.-Jun.	Feb.-Jul.	Feb.-Jul.	Jan.-Jun.	Jan.-Jun.	Mar.-Jul.	Feb.-Jul.	Jan.-Jul.
BLUEGRASS, CANADIAN (Poa compressa)	Jun.-Jul.	N May-Jun.	Jun.-Jul.	Jun.-Jul.	N Jun.-Jul.	N Jun.-Jul.	Jun.-Jul.	Jun.-Jul.	N Jun.-Jul.
BLUEGRASS, KENTUCKY (Poa pratensis) †	Jun.-Jul. •	N May-Jun. •	Jun.-Jul. •	Jun.-Jul. •	N Apr.-Jun. •	N Apr.-Jun. •	Jun.-Jul. •	Jun.-Jul. •	May-Jul. •
BROME, CALIFORNIA (Bromus carinatus)						S May-Jun.			May-Jun.
BROME, HUNGARIAN (Bromus inermis) †			May-Jun. •	Jun.-Jul. •	N May-Jun. •	N May-Jun. •	Jun.-Jul. •	Jun.-Jul. •	May-Jul. •
BROME, SMOOTH (Bromus inermis) †			May-Jun. •	Jun.-Jul. •	N May-Jun. •	N May-Jun. •	Jun.-Jul. •	Jun.-Jul. •	May-Jul. •
CANARY GRASS, REED (Phalaris arundinacea)	Jun.-Jul.		Jun.-Jul.	Jun.-Jul.	N May-Jun. •	N Jun.-Jul. •	Jun.-Jul.	Jun.-Jul.	N Jun.-Jul. •
CHEAT GRASS (Bromus secalinus)	Jun.-Jul.	May-Jun.	Jun.-Jul.	Jun.-Jul.	May-Jun.	May-Jun.	Jun.-Jul.	Jun.-Jul.	May-Jun.
CORN (Zea mays)	Jul.-Aug.	Jun.-Sep.	Jul.-Aug.	Jul.-Aug.	Jun.-Sep.	Jun.-Sep.	Jul.-Aug.	Jul.-Aug.	Jun.-Sep.
CREEPING BENT (Agrostis palustris)	Jun.-Jul.		Jun.-Jul.			Jun.-Jul.	NW Jun.-Jul.	Jun.-Jul.	N Jun.-Jul.
FESCUE, MEADOW (Festuca elatior)	May-Jun.	N May-Jun. •	May-Jun. •	May-Jun. •	N May-Jun. •	May-Jul. •	Jun.-Jul.	May-Jul. •	May-Jul. •
GRAMA GRASS (Bouteloua spp.)				Jun.-Sep.	Jun.-Jul.	Jun.-Aug.	Jun.-Sep.		
JOHNSON GRASS (Sorghum halepense)	Jun.-Sep.	Jun.-Oct. •	Jun.-Sep. •	Jun.-Oct.	Jun.-Oct. •	Jun.-Oct.	SW Jul.-Sep.		S Jun.-Oct. •
JUNE GRASS (Poa pratensis) †	Jun.-Jul. •	N May-Jun. •	Jun.-Jul. •	Jun.-Jul. •	N Apr.-Jun. •	N Apr.-Jun. •	Jun.-Jul. •	Jun.-Jul. •	May-Jul. •
JUNE GRASS, WESTERN (Koeleria cristata)	Jun.-Jul.	SW Jun.-Jul.	Jun.-Jul.	Jun.-Jul.	N May-Jun.	Jun.-Jul.	Jun.-Jul.	Jun.-Jul.	Jun.-Jul.
OAT GRASS, TALL (Arrhenatherum elatius)	Jun.-Jul.	N May-Jun.	May-Jul.		May-Jul.			Jun.-Jul.	N May-Jul.
OATS, CULTIVATED (Avena sativa)	May-Jun.	Apr.-May	May-Jun.	May-Jun.	May-Jun.	May-Jul.	May-Jul.	May-Jul.	May-Jul.

GRASSES (continued)

	COMMON/SCIENTIFIC NAME	ZONE 1	ZONE 2	ZONE 3	ZONE 4	ZONE 5	ZONE 6	ZONE 7	ZONE 8	ZONE 9
GRASSES	OATS, WILD (Avena fatua)	May-Jun.		May-Jun.	N May-Jun.		Apr.-Jun.	May-Jun.	May-Jun.	May-Jul. •
	ORCHARD GRASS (Dactylis glomerata)	May-Jul. •	May-Jun. •	May-Jun. •	May-Jun. •	N May	N May-Jul. •	May-Jul. •	May-Jul. •	May-Jul. •
	QUACK GRASS (Agropyron repens)	Jun.-Jul.		Jun.-Jul.	Jun.-Jul. •	N Jun.-Jul.	N Jun.-Aug.	Jun.-Aug.	Jun.-Aug. •	N Jun.-Aug.
	REDTOP (Agrostis alba)	Jun.-Jul. •	N Jun.-Jul. •	Jun.-Jul. •	Jun.-Aug. •	N Jun.-Jul. •	N Jun.-Aug. •	Jun.-Aug. •	Jun.-Aug. •	N Jun.-Aug. •
	RYE, ALKALI (Elymus triticoides)						Jun.-Jul.	Jun.-Jul.	Jun.-Jul.	Jun.-Jul.
	RYE, CULTIVATED (Secale cereale)	May-Jun.	Apr.-May	May-Jun.	May-Jun.-	Apr.-May	Apr.-Jun.	May-Jun.	May-Jun.	Apr.-Jun.
	RYE, GIANT WILD (Slymus condensatus)								Jun.-Aug. •	Jun.-Aug.
	RYE GRASS, ITALIAN (Lolium multiflorum)	May-Aug.	N May-Jul. •	May-Jun. •	May-Jul. •	May-Jun.	N May-Aug. •	Jun.-Aug. •	Jun.-Aug. •	May-Aug. •
	RYE GRASS, PERENNIAL (Lolium perenne)	May-Aug.	N May-Jul. •	May-Jun. •	May-Jul. •	May-Jun.	N May-Aug. •	Jun.-Aug. •	Jun.-Aug. •	May-Aug. •
	SALT GRASS (Distichlis spicata)	Jun.-Jul.	May-Jun.		May-Jun.	May-Jun.	May-Jun.	Jun.-Jul.	Jun.-Jul.	May-Jul. •
	SUDAN GRASS (Sorghum vulgare var. sudanesis) †		Jul.-Sep.	S Jul.-Sep.		Jul.-Sep.	Jul.-Sep.			Jul.-Sep.
	SORGHUM (Sorghum vulgare) †		Jul.-Sep.	S Jul.-Sep.		Jul.-Sep.	Jul.-Sep.			Jul.-Sep.
	SWEET VERNAL GRASS (Anthoxanthum odoratum)	May-Jun.	N May-Jun. •						W May-Jun. •	W May-Jun.
	TIMOTHY (Phleum pratense)	Jun.-Jul. •	N Jun.-Jul. •	Jun.-Jul. •	Jul. •	Jun.-Jul.	Jun.-Aug. •	Jul.-Aug. •	Jun.-Aug. •	Jun.-Jul. •
	VELVET GRASS (Holcus lanatus)	Jun.-Aug.	Jun.-Aug.	S Jun.-Aug.					Jun.-Aug. •	Jun.-Aug.
	WHEAT, CULTIVATED (Triticum aestivum)	May-Jul.	May-Jun.	May-Jul.	May-Jul.	May-Jun.	May-Jul.	Jun.-Jul.	May-Jul.	May-Jul.
	WHEAT GRASS, CRESTED (Agropyron cristatum)			Jun.-Jul.	Jun.-Jul.		Jun.-Aug.	Jun.-Aug.		Jun.-Aug.
	WHEAT GRASS, WESTERN (Agropyron smithii)			Jun.-Jul.	Jun.-Jul. •	N Jun.-Jul. •	Jun.-Aug. •	Jun.-Aug. •	Jun.-Aug. •	Jun.-Aug.

† This plant is also known by another name; consult Synonomous Names Cross Reference for other name(s).
N, S, E, W Indicates this plant is found in the Northern, Southern, Eastern, or Western region of that particular zone.
• Primary allergic significance due to either volume of pollen produced, potency of pollen produced, or a combination of the two.

HAY FEVER PLANTS ARRANGED IN PHYLOGENETIC ORDER

1. **PINACEAE: PINE FAMILY**
   - Abies grandis (White Fir)
   - Cedrus deodara (Deodara Cedar)
   - Cupressus arizonica (Arizona Cypress)
   - Cupressus macrocarpa (Monterey Cypress)
   - Juniperus californica (Calif. Juniper)
   - Juniperus deppeana (Alligator Juniper)
   - Juniperus monosperma (Oneseed Juniper)
   - Juniperus occidentalis (West. Juniper)
   - Juniperus osteosperma (Utah Juniper)
   - Juniperus pinchotii (Redberry Juniper)
   - Juniperus sabinoides (Mountain Cedar)
   - Juniperus scopulorum (Rocky Mt. Juniper)
   - Juniperus virginiana (Red Cedar)
   - Larix spp. (Tamarack)
   - Libocedrus decurrens (Incense Cedar)
   - Picea pungens (Blue Spruce)
   - Picea rubens (Red Spruce)
   - Picea sitchensis (Sitka Spruce)
   - Pinus contorta (Lodgepole Pine)
   - Pinus echinata (Shortleaf Pine)
   - Pinus edulis (Pinyon Pine)
   - Pinus elliotti (Slash Pine)
   - Pinus nigra (Austrian Pine)
   - Pinus palustris (Longleaf Pine)
   - Pinus ponderosa (Ponderosa Pine)
   - Pinus resinosa (Red Pine)
   - Pinus strobus (White Pine)
   - Pinus sylvestris (Scotch Pine)
   - Pinus taeda (Loblolly Pine)
   - Pinus virginiana (Virginia Pine)
   - Pseudotsuga taxifolia (Douglas Fir)
   - Sequoia spp. (Redwood)
   - Taxodium distichum (Bald Cypress)
   - Thuja orientalis (Arbor Vitae)
   - Tsuga spp. (Hemlock)

2. **TAXACEAE: YEW FAMILY**
   - Taxus spp. (Yew)

3. **GRAMINEAE: GRASS FAMILY**

   TRIBE I—Bambuseae
   - Arundinaria gigantea (Cane)
   - Bromus inermis (Smooth Brome)
   - Bromus secalinus (Chess)
   - Bromus carinatus (Calif. Brome)
   - Bromus rigidus (Ringut)

   TRIBE II—Festeuceae
   - Festuca elatior (Meadow Fescue)
   - Festuca rubra (Red Fescue)
   - Festuca ovina (Sheep Fescue)
   - Poa annua (Annual Blue Grass)
   - Poa compressa (Canada Blue Grass)
   - Poa pratensis (Kentucky Blue Grass)
   - Poa trivialis (Rough Blue Grass)
   - Eragrostis reptans (Creeping Love Grass)
   - Eragrostis ciliianensis (Stink Grass)
   - Distichlis spicata (Seashore Salt Grass)
   - Distichlis stricta (Inland Salt Grass)
   - Dactylis glomerata (Orchard Grass)

   TRIBE III—Hordeae
   - Agropyron repens (Quack Grass)
   - Agropyron smithii (West. Wheat Grass)
   - Agropyron cristatum (Crested Wheat Grass)
   - Agropyron trachycaulum (Bearded Wheat Grass)
   - Triticum aestivum (Cultivated Wheat)
   - Secale cereale (Cultivated Rye)
   - Elymus condensatus (Giant Wild Rye)
   - Elymus triticoides (Alkali Rye)
   - Hordeum vulgare (Barley)
   - Lolium perenne (Perennial Rye Grass)
   - Lolium multiflorum (Italian Rye Grass)
   - Lolium temulentum (Darnel Rye Grass)

   TRIBE IV—Aveneae
   - Koeleria cristata (Western June Grass)
   - Avena barbata (Slender Wild Oat)
   - Avena fatua (Wild Oats)
   - Avena sativa (Cultivated Oats)
   - Arrhenatherum elatius (Tall Oat Grass)
   - Holcus lanatus (Velvet Grass)

   TRIBE V—Agrostideae
   - Agrostis alba (Redtop)
   - Agrostis tenuis (Bent Grass)
   - Phleum pratense (Timothy)

   TRIBE VI—Chlorideae
   - Cynodon dactylon (Bermuda Grass)
   - Bouteloua curtipendula (Side-Oat-Grama)
   - Bouteloua gracilis (Blue Gramma)
   - Buchloe dactyloides (Buffalo Grass)

   TRIBE VII—Phalarideae
   - Anthoxanthum odoratum (Sweet Vernal Grass)
   - Phalaris canariensis (Canary Grass)
   - Phalaris arundinacea (Reed Canary Grass)

   TRIBE VIII—Oryzeae
   - Oryza sativa (Rice)

   TRIBE IX—Zizanieae
   - Zizania aquatica (Wild Rice)

   TRIBE X—Paniceae
   - Digitaria sanguinalis (Crab Grass)
   - Paspalum dilatatum (Dallis Grass)
   - Echinochloa crusgalli (Barnyard Grass)
   - Setaria glauca (Yellow Foxtail)

   TRIBE XI—Andropogoneae
   - Andropogon gerardi (Bib Blue Stem)
   - Sorghum halepense (Johnson Grass)
   - Sorghum sudanense (Sudan Grass)
   - Sorghum vulgare (Cane)
   - Sorgastrum nutans (Indian Grass)

   TRIBE XII—Tripsaceae
   - Tripsacum dactyloides (Gama Grass)
   - Zea mays (Corn)

4. **PALMACEAE: PALM FAMILY**
   - Cocos nucefera (Cocoanut Palm)
   - Phoenix dactylifera (Date Palm)
   - Phoenix canariensis (Ornamental Palm)

5. **SALICACEAE: WILLOW FAMILY**
   - Populus alba (White Poplar)
   - Populus balsamifera (Balsam Poplar)
   - Populus deltoides (East. Cottonwood)
   - Populus fremontii (Ariz. Cottonwood)
   - Populus nigra italica (Lombardy Poplar)
   - Populus sargentii (West. Cottonwood)
   - Populus tremuloides (Quaking Aspen)
   - Populus trichocarpa (Black Cottonwood)
   - Populus wislizenii (Rio Grande Cottonwood)
   - Salix discolor (Pussy Willow)
   - Salix nigra (Black Willow)

6. **JUGLANDACEAE: WALNUT FAMILY**
   - Carya cordiformis (Bitternut Hickory)
   - Carya glabra (Pignut Hickory)
   - Carya illinoensis (Pecan)
   - Carya laciniosa (Shellbark Hickory)
   - Carya ovata (Shagbark Hickory)
   - Carya tomentosa (White Hickory)
   - Juglans californica (Calif. Blk. Walnut)
   - Juglans cinerea (Butternut)
   - Juglans nigra (Black Walnut)
   - Juglans regia (English Walnut)
   - Juglans rupestris (Mexican Walnut)

7. **BETULACEAE: BIRCH FAMILY**
   - Alnus rhombifolia (White Alder)
   - Alnus rubra (Red Alder)
   - Alnus rugosa (Smooth Alder)
   - Alnus tenuifolia (Thinleaf Alder)
   - Betula alleghaniensis (Yellow Birch)
   - Betula lenta (Sweet Birch)
   - Betula nigra (River Birch)
   - Betula occidentalis (Water Birch)
   - Betula papyrifera (Paper Birch)
   - Betula populifolia (White Birch)
   - Carpinus caroliniana (Hop-Hornbeam)
   - Corylus americana (Hazelnut)
   - Corylus californica (Calif. Hazelnut)
   - Ostrya virginiana (Ironwood)

8. **FAGACEAE: BEECH FAMILY**
   - Castanea spp. (Chestnut)
   - Fagus grandifolia (American Beech)
   - Quercus agrifolia (Calif. Live Oak)
   - Quercus alba (White Oak)
   - Quercus chrysolepsis (Canyon Live Oak)
   - Quercus coccinea (Scarlet Oak)
   - Quercus douglasii (Blue Oak)
   - Quercus dumosa (Calif. Scrub Oak)
   - Quercus falcata (Southern Red Oak)
   - Quercus gambelii (Gambel's Oak)
   - Quercus garryana (Western White Oak)
   - Quercus kelloggii (Calif. Black Oak)
   - Quercus lobata (Calif. White Oak)
   - Quercus macrocarpa (Bur Oak)
   - Quercus marilandica (Blackjack Oak)
   - Quercus nigra (Water Oak)
   - Quercus palustris (Pin Oak)
   - Quercus phellos (Willow Oak)
   - Quercus prinoides (Dwarf Chinkapin Oak)
   - Quercus prinus (Chestnut Oak)
   - Quercus rubra (Red Oak)
   - Quercus stellata (Post Oak)
   - Quercus stellata var. margaretta (Dwarf Post)
   - Quercus velutina (Black Oak)
   - Quercus virginiana (Live Oak)

9. **ULMACEAE: ELM FAMILY**
   - Celtis occidentalis (Hackberry)
   - Ulmus alata (Winged Elm)
   - Ulmus americana (American Elm)
   - Ulmus crassifolia (Cedar Elm)
   - Ulmus parvifolia (Fall Blooming Elm)
   - Ulmus pumila (Chinese Elm)
   - Ulmus rubra (Slippery Elm)

10. **MORACEAE: MULBERRY FAMILY**
    - Broussonetia papyrifera (Paper Mulberry)
    - Maclura pomifera (Osage Orange)
    - Morus alba (White Mulberry)
    - Morus rubra (Red Mulberry)

11. **URTICACEAE: NETTLE FAMILY**
    - Urtica spp. (Nettle)

12. **POLYGONACEAE: BUCKWHEAT FAMILY**
    - Rumex acetosella (Sheep Sorrel)
    - Rumex altissimus (Tall Dock)
    - Rumex crispus (Yellow Dock)
    - Rumex hymenosepalus (Wild Rhubarb)
    - Rumex mexicanus (White Dock)
    - Rumex obtusifolia (Bitter Dock)

Continued

13. **CHENOPODIACEAE: GOOSEFOOT FAMILY**
- Allenrolfea occidentalis (Iodine Bush)
- Atriplex argentea (Silverscale)
- Atriplex bracteosa (Bractscale)
- Atriplex brewerii (Coast Saltbush)
- Atriplex canescens (Wingscale)
- Atriplex confertifolia (Shadescale)
- Atriplex lentiformis (Lenscale)
- Atriplex patula hastata (Spearscale)
- Atriplex polycarpa (Allscale)
- Atriplex rosea (Redscale)
- Atriplex wrightii (Annual Saltbush)
- Bassia hyssopifolia (Bassia)
- Beta vulgaris (Beet)
- Chenopodium album (Lamb's Quarters)
- Chenopodium ambrosioides (Mexican Tea)
- Chenopodium anthelmenticum (Wormseed)
- Chenopodium botrys (Jerusalem Oak)
- Chenopodium murale (Nettle-leaved Goosefoot)
- Chenopodium paganum (Summer Lamb's Quarters)
- Eurotia lanata (Winter Fat)
- Kochia scoparia (Firebush)
- Salicornia ambigua (Pickleweed)
- Salsola kali tenuifolia (Russian Thistle)
- Sarcobatus vermiculatus (Greasewood)
- Suaeda (Sea Blite)

14. **AMARANTHACEAE: AMARANTH FAMILY**
- Acnida tamariscina (Western Water Hemp)
- Amaranthus hybridus (Green Amaranth)
- Amaranthus palmeri (Carelessweed)
- Amaranthus retroflexus (Rough Pigweed)
- Amaranthus spinosus (Spiny Pigweed)

15. **MAGNOLIACEAE: MAGNOLIA FAMILY**
- Magnolia spp. (Magnolia)

16. **HAMMELIDACEAE: WITCH HAZEL FAMILY**
- Liquidambar styraciflua (Sweetgum)

17. **PLATANACEAE: PLANETREE FAMILY**
- Platanus acerifolia (London Planetree)
- Platanus occidentalis (Sycamore)
- Platanus racemosa (Calif. Sycamore)

18. **ROSACEAE: ROSE FAMILY**
- Malus spp. (Apple)
- Prunus spp. (Cherry, Peach, Apricot, Plum)
- Rosa spp. (Rose)

19. **LEGUMINOSAE: PEA FAMILY**
- Acacia spp.
- Cercidium spp. (Paloverde)
- Medicago sativa (Alfalfa)
- Melilotus spp. (Sweet Clover)
- Prosopis spp. (Mesquite)
- Robinia pseudoacacia (Black Locust)
- Trifolium pratense (Red Clover)
- Trifolium repens (White Clover)
- Vicia spp. (Vetch)

20. **RUTACEAE: RUE FAMILY**
- Citrus spp. (Orange, Lime, Lemon)

21. **SIMAROUBACEAE: QUASSIA FAMILY**
- Ailanthus altissima (Tree-of-Heaven)

22. **EUPHORBIACEAE: SPURGE FAMILY**
- Sapium sebiferum (Chinese Tallow)

23. **ANACARDIACEAE: SUMAC FAMILY**
- Rhus capallina (Sumac)
- Schinus molle (Peppertree)

24. **ACERACEAE: MAPLE FAMILY**
- Acer macrophyllum (Coast Maple)
- Acer regundo (Box Elder)
- Acer rubrum (Red Maple)
- Acer saccharinum (Soft Maple)
- Acer saccharum (Sugar Maple)

25. **HIPPOCASTANACEAE: HORSE CHESTNUT FAMILY**
- Aesculus spp. (Buckeye)

26. **TILIACEAE: LINDEN FAMILY**
- Tilia spp. (Basswood; Linden)

27. **TAMARICACEAE: TAMARISK FAMILY**
- Tamarix gallica (Salt Cedar)

28. **ELAEAGNACEAE: RUSSIAN OLIVE FAMILY**
- Elaeagnus angustifolia (Russian Olive)

29. **MYRTACEAE: MYRTLE FAMILY**
- Eucalyptus spp.

30. **CORNACEAE: DOGWOOD FAMILY**
- Cornus spp. (Dogwood)
- Nyssa sylvatica (Black Gum)

31. **OLEACEAE: OLIVE FAMILY**
- Fraxinus americana (White Ash)
- Fraxinus pennsylvanica (Red or Green Ash)
- Fraxinus quadrangulata (Blue Ash)
- Fraxinus oregona (Oregon Ash)
- Fraxinus velutina (Arizona Ash)
- Ligustrum spp. (Privet)
- Olea europea (Olive)

32. **PLANTAGINACEAE: PLANTAIN FAMILY**
- Plantago lanceolata (English Plantain)
- Plantago major (Common Plantain)

33. **COMPOSITAE: COMPOSITE FAMILY**

TRIBE I—Astereae
- Baccharis spp. (Groundsel Tree)
- Chrysothamnus nauseous (Rabbitbrush)
- Gutierrezia dracunculoides (Broomweed)
- Solidago spp. (Goldenrod)
- Haplopappus ciliatus (Prionopsis)
- Aster spp. (Aster)

TRIBE II—Heliantheae
- Iva angustifolia (Narrowleaf Marsh Elder)
- Iva axillaris (Povertyweed)
- Iva ciliata (Rough Marsh Elder)
- Iva xanthifolia (Burweed Marsh Elder)
- Ambrosia aptera (West. Giant Ragweed)
- Ambrosia artemisiifolia (Short Ragweed)
- Ambrosia bidentata (Southern Ragweed)
- Ambrosia coronopifolia (West. Ragweed)
- Ambrosia trifida (Giant Ragweed)
- Franseria acanthicarpa (False Ragweed)
- Franseria ambrosioides (Canyon Ragweed)
- Franseria bipinnatifida (Beach Sandbur)
- Franseria chamissonis (Silver Beachwood)
- Franseria deltoidea (Rabbit Bush)
- Franseria discolor (Low Ragweed)
- Franseria dumosa (Desert Ragweed)
- Franseria tenuifolia (Slender Ragweed)
- Franseria tomentosa (Woolly Ragweed)
- Xanthium commune (Cocklebur)
- Xanthium spinosum (Spiny Cocklebur)
- Helianthus spp. (Sunflower)
- Coreopsis spp.
- Cosmos spp.

TRIBE III—Helenieae
- Tagetes (Marigold)

TRIBE IV—Anthemideae
- Achillea millefolium (Yarrow)
- Anthemis cotula (Dog Fennel)
- Chrysanthemum spp. (Daisy)
- Artemisia absinthium (Common Wormwood)
- Artemisia annua (Annual Wormwood)
- Artemisia biennis (Biennial Wormwood)
- Artemisia californica (Coast Sage)
- Artemisia campestris (Sagewort)
- Artemisia dracunculus (Indian Hair Tonic)
- Artemisia filifolia (Sand Sage)
- Artemisia frigida (Carpet Sage)
- Artemisia gnaphalodes (Prairie Sage)
- Artemisia heterophylla (California Mugwort)
- Artemisia ludoviciana (Dark-leaved Mugwort)
- Artemisia tridentata (Sagebrush)
- Artemisia vulgaris (Common Mugwort)

TRIBE V—Cichorieae
- Taraxacum officinale (Dandelion)

Synonymous Name Cross Reference

Genus/species	Common Names
Acer saccharinum	Soft maple, silver maple
Acer saccharum	Sugar maple, hard maple
Amaranthus palmeri	Carelessweed, Palmer's amaranth
Amaranthus retroflexus	Rough pigweed, redroot pigweed
Ambrosia artemisifolia, Ambrosia elatior	Short ragweed, low ragweed, dwarf ragweed, common ragweed
Ambrosia coronopifolia, Ambrosia psilostachya	Western ragweed
Artemisia dracunculus	Dragon sage, green sage, Indian hair tonic
Artemisia frigida	Pasture sage, carpet sage
Baccharis spp.	Groundsel tree, baccharis, ranch willow, grandfather's beard
Betula nigra	River birch, red birch
Bromus inermis	Hungarian brome, smooth brome
Carya illinoensis, Hicoria pecan	Pecan
Iva ciliata	Rough marshelder, true marshelder
Juniperus pinchotii	Redberry juniper, Pinchot cedar, cherrystone juniper
Juniperus sabinoides, Juniperus asheii	Mountain cedar
Kochia scoparia	Kochia, firebush, burning bush, summer cypress
Ligustrum spp.	Ligustrum, privet
Poa pratensis	Kentucky blue grass, June grass
Populus deltoides	Eastern cottonwood, common cottonwood
Populus fremontii	Arizona cottonwood, fremont poplar
Rumex acetosella	Sheep sorrel, sour dock
Salsola Kali tenuifolia	Russian thistle, tumbleweed
Sorghum Vulgare	Sudan grass, sorghum
Ulmus crassifolia	Fall blooming elm, cedar elm, basket elm
Xanthium commune, Xanthium pennsylvanicum	Cocklebur

Bibliography

Baerg HJ. *How to Know the Western Trees*. Dubuque, IA: William C. Brown, 1955.

Coker WC, Totten HR. *Trees of the Southeastern States*. Durham, NC: The University of North Carolina Press, 1937.

Davis RJ. *Flora of Idaho*. Dubuque, IA: William C. Brown, 1952.

Emerson AI, Weed CM. *Our Trees—How to Know Them*. Garden City, NY: Garden City Publishing Co., 1946.

Featherly HI. *Manual of the Grasses of Oklahoma*. Stillwater, OK: Oklahoma Agricultural and Mechanical College, 1946.

Featherly HI. *Trees of Oklahoma*. Oklahoma City, OK: Forestry Division State Board of Agriculture, 1975.

Featherly HI. *Silvics of Forest Trees of the United States*. Washington, DC: US Government Printing Office, 1965.

Featherly HI. Grass, *The Yearbook of Agriculture*. Washington, DC: US Government Printing Office, 1948.

Harrar ES, Harrar JG. *Guide to Southern Trees*. New York: McGraw-Hill, 1946.
Harrington HD. *Manual of the Plants of Colorado*. Denver, CO: Alan Swallow, 1954, 1964.
Jacques HE. *How to Know the Weeds*. Dubuque, IA: William C. Brown, 1959.
Jacques HE, Miller HA. *How to Know the Trees*. Dubuque, IA: William C. Brown, 1941, 1972.
Kearney TH, Peebles RH: *Arizona Flora*. Berkeley and Los Angeles: University of California Press, 1964.
Levetin E, Buck P: Hayfever Plants in Oklahoma. *Ann Allerg* 1980;45.
Little EL Jr. *Check List of Native and Naturalized Trees of the United States*. Washington, DC: US Government Printing Office, 1953.
Little EL Jr. Nebraska Weeds, Bulletin No. 101-R, Revised Summer 1962, Lincoln, NE: Weed and Seed Division, Department of Agriculture and Inspection, 1962.
Pohl RW: *How to Know the Grasses*. Dubuque, IA: William C. Brown, 1954, 1968.
Preston RJ Jr. *Rocky Mountain Trees*. Ames, IA: The Iowa State College Press, 1940.
Robbins WW, Bellue MK, Ball, WS. *Weeds of California*. Sacramento, CA: California State Department of Agriculture, 1951.
Sargent CS. *Manual of the Trees of North America*. Boston, New York: The Riverside Press, Cambridge, 1905, 1922, 1933.
Stemen TR, Myers WS. *Oklahoma Flora*. Oklahoma City, OK: Harlow, 1937.
Steyermark JA. *Flora of Missouri*. Ames, IA: The Iowa State University Press.
Steyermark JA. *Spring Flora of Missouri*. Fulton, MO: The Ovid Bell Press, 1940.
Steyermark JA: *Texas Plants, A Checklist and Ecological Summary*. College Station, TX: Texas Agricultural Extension Service, Texas A&M University, 1969.
Van Dersal WR. *Native Woody Plants of the United States*. Washington, DC: United States Government Printing Office, 1938.
Van Dersal WR. *Weeds of the North Central States*. Publication No. 36, Circular 718, Urbana, IL: University of Illinois Agricultural Experiment Station, 1954.
Van Dersal WR. *Weeds of the Southern United States*. College Station, TX: Texas Agricultural Extension Service, Texas A&M University.
Wodehouse RP. *Pollen Grains*. New York: Hafner, 1965.

· Index ·

(Italic page numbers indicate a table or figure.)